TCHマネジメントとリハビリトレーニングで治す顎関節症

TCH Management and Rehabilitation Training Methods for TMD

編著　木野 孔司　Koji Kino
著　　佐藤 文明　Fumiaki Sato
　　　儀武 啓幸　Hiroyuki Yoshitake
　　　和気 裕之　Hiroyuki Wake
監訳　Nguyen Gia Kieu Ngan

日本発 木野メソッドによるアプローチ

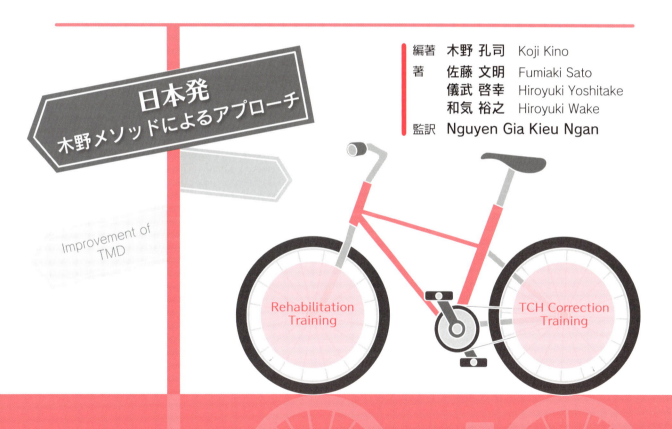

Improvement of TMD

Rehabilitation Training

TCH Correction Training

医歯薬出版株式会社

This book was originally published in Japanese
under the title of :
TCH MANEJIMENTO TO RIHABIRI-TORENINGU DE NAOSU GAKUKANSETSUSHO
—NIHON-HATSU KINO-MESODDO NIYORU APUROCHI—
(TCH Management and Rehabilitation Training Methods for TMD)

Editors :
KINO, Koji et al.

KINO, Koji
  Kino TMJ Institute

© 2019 1st ed.

ISHIYAKU PUBLISHERS, INC.
  7-10, Honkomagome 1 chome, Bunkyo-ku,
  Tokyo 113-8612, Japan

Contributors

木野 孔司　Koji Kino

1976年　東京医科歯科大学歯学部卒業
1980年　東京医科歯科大学大学院歯学研究科修了，歯学博士
1981年　東京医科歯科大学歯学部口腔外科学第一講座助手
2000年　東京医科歯科大学歯学部助教授，附属病院顎関節治療部部長
2015年　木野顎関節研究所所長，鶴見大学臨床教授，東京医科歯科大学大学院口腔顔面痛制御学分野非常勤講師

日本顎関節学会専門医・指導医

1976	D.D.S., Tokyo Medical and Dental University
1980	Ph.D., Tokyo Medical and Dental University
1981	Research Associate, Tokyo Medical and Dental University, The First Department of Oral and Maxillofacial Surgery
2000	Director and Associate Professor, Tokyo Medical and Dental University, Temporomandibular Joint Clinic
2015-	Director, Kino TMJ Research Institute
Clinical Professor, Tsurumi University
Part-time Lecturer, Tokyo Medical and Dental University

Certified Specialist and Supervisor, The Japanese Society for Temporomandibular Joint

儀武 啓幸　Hiroyuki Yoshitake

1995年　鶴見大学歯学部卒業
1995年　東京医科歯科大学大学院口腔外科学第一講座専攻生
2000年　東京医科歯科大学大学院歯学研究科修了，博士（歯学）
　　　　東京厚生年金病院歯科口腔外科医員
2001年　東京医科歯科大学大学院顎顔面外科学分野医員
2006年　東京医科歯科大学大学院顎顔面外科学分野助教
2007年　鶴見大学歯学部薬理学講座非常勤講師

日本顎関節学会専門医・指導医

1995	D.D.S., Tsurumi University, School of Dental Medicine
1995	Graduate Student, Tokyo Medical and Dental University, The First Department of Oral and Maxillofacial Surgery
2000	Ph.D., Tokyo Medical and Dental University
2001	Clinical Fellow, Tokyo Medical and Dental University, Department of Oral and Maxillofacial Surgery
2006-	Research Associate, Tokyo Medical and Dental University, Department of Oral and Maxillofacial Surgery
2007-	Part-time Lecturer, Tsurumi University

Certified Specialist and Supervisor, The Japanese Society for Temporomandibular Joint
International Member, American Society of Temporomandibular Joint Surgeons
Founding Member, Japanese Society of Temporomandibular Joint Surgeons

佐藤 文明　Fumiaki Sato

1989年　北海道大学歯学部卒業
1989年　東京医科歯科大学歯学部口腔外科学第一講座専攻生
1993年　佐藤歯科医院　開設（東京都台東区）
2004年　東京医科歯科大学大学院顎顔面外科学分野非常勤講師
2007年　博士（歯学）（東京医科歯科大学）
2016年　佐藤歯科医院　今戸クリニック　開設（東京都台東区）

日本顎関節学会専門医・指導医，日本口腔インプラント学会専門医

1989	D.D.S., Hokkaido University, School of Dental Medicine
1989	Graduate Student, Tokyo Medical and Dental University, The First Department of Oral and Maxillofacial Surgery
1993	Director, Sato Dental Clinic (Tokyo)
2004-	Part-time Lecturer, Tokyo Medical and Dental University
2007	Ph.D., Tokyo Medical and Dental University
2016-	Director, Sato Dental Office Imado Clinic (Tokyo)

Certified Specialist and Supervisor, The Japanese Society for Temporomandibular Joint
Certified Specialist, The Japanese Society of Dental Implantology

和気 裕之　Hiroyuki Wake

1978年　日本大学松戸歯学部卒業
1978年　東京医科歯科大学歯学部口腔外科学第一講座専攻生
1981年　みどり小児歯科　開設（横浜市青葉区）
2016年　日本顎関節学会副理事長（～2018年）

日本大学客員教授，昭和大学客員教授，神奈川歯科大学客員教授，東京医科歯科大学臨床教授，北海道大学客員臨床教授，長崎大学非常勤講師
日本顎関節学会専門医・指導医，日本口腔顔面痛学会専門医・指導医，日本歯科心身医学会代議員

1978	D.D.S, Nihon University School of Dentistry at Matsudo
1978	Graduate Student, Tokyo Medical and Dental University, The First Department of Oral and Maxillofacial Surgery
1981-	Director, Midori Pediatric Dental Clinic (Yokohama-city)
1999	Ph.D., Tokyo Medical and Dental University
2016-2018	Vice Chief Director, The Japanese Society for Temporomandibular Joint

Visiting Professor, Nihon University; Showa University; Kanagawa Dental College
Clinical Professor, Tokyo Medical and Dental University
Visiting Clinical Professor, Hokkaido University
Part-time Lecturer, Nagasaki University
Certified Specialist and Supervisor, Japanese Society for Temporomandibular Joint; Japanese Society of Orofacial Pain
Representative, Japanese Society of Psychosomatic Dentistry

【translation supervisor】
Nguyen Gia Kieu Ngan　グイン ヤー キエウ ガン

2013年　フエ医科薬科大学歯学部卒業
2013年　フエ医科薬科大学歯学部講師
2015年　東京医科歯科大学口腔顔面痛制御学分野大学院生

日本顎関節学会会員

2013	D.D.S, Hue University of Medicine and Pharmacy, Faculty of Odonto-Stomatology
2013	Lecturer, Hue University of Medicine and Pharmacy, Faculty of Odonto-Stomatology
2015-	Ph.D. Student, Tokyo Medical and Dental University

Member, The Japanese Society for Temporomandibular Joint

Preface

　顎関節症の病因としてTCH（Tooth Contacting Habit：上下歯列接触癖）の概念を公表してから，10年以上が経過した．TCHが病因であることを発見した当初は，それを是正する有効な手法を見出せず試行錯誤を続けたが，ある時，応用心理学の領域で行われている「習慣逆転法」と呼ばれる行動療法の存在を知った．これをTCHに応用するには3年ほど工夫を要したものの，現在ではTCH是正訓練の手法は完成したと言えるだろう．

　さらに，顎関節症の病態に対する治療として「リハビリトレーニング」と称した運動療法を，病因治療としてのTCH是正訓練と並行して行うことによって，それまで難治性とされていた顎関節症を効果的に改善できるようになった．そのうえ，患者自身がTCHの有無をチェックして顎関節症の再発を防止することも可能となり，「顎関節症は再発を繰り返す慢性疾患である」という難病感は払拭されてきている．

　TCH是正訓練とリハビリトレーニングについては，すでにそれぞれ書籍を上梓しているが，顎関節症治療においては両者を自転車の両輪のように並行して進めることが重要であるため，本書ではその治療コンセプトを「木野メソッド」としてまとめた．病因と病態に対する診断，治療のポイントをわかりやすく解説するよう努め，実践的な顎関節症治療の入門書として読んでいただけると思う．

　また，本書では新しい試みとして，全編にわたって英語を併記した．TCH是正訓練は非侵襲的かつ効果の高い治療法だが，残念ながら海外ではまだあまり知られていない．しかし最近，世界各地からの見学者や留学生から，「日本にはこんなに優れた治療法があったのか！」と，TCH是正訓練の習得に興味を示してもらえることが多くなった．アジア諸国を含めた多くの国では，歯科関係の書物の多くが英語で書かれており，英語を併記することで海外の歯科医がわれわれの治療コンセプトを理解し，母国で臨床応用してくれることを期待している．

　さらに日本でも，海外からの観光客の増加に伴い，顎関節症で来院する外国人患者を診る機会もあると思われる．そのような時に，英語が併記された本書をチェアサイドで活用していただきたい．付録の問診票の書式も英語版を用意しており，外国人患者の診療をスムーズに進める助けになると思われる．

　本書が多くの歯科医に利用されることで，世界の顎関節症治療が大きく変化し，顎関節症に苦しむ患者さんがいなくなることを願っている．

2019年6月

木野孔司

More than ten years have passed since we officially announced the concept of Tooth Contacting Habit (TCH) as an etiology of temporomandibular disorder (TMD). In those days when we found out that TCH might cause TMD, finding effective modalities to correct TCH was thoroughly challenging, however, we had kept practicing trial process. But on one occasion, I learned a behavioral therapy called "habit reversal method" which is utilized in the field of applied psychology. It took approximately three years to modify this method before applying it to TCH, and it can be said that the method of TCH correction training has been completely established.

In addition, a therapeutic exercise named "rehabilitation training" is performed to reduce the symptoms of TMD in parallel with TCH correction training as etiological treatment. This combination has effectively improved TMD which had been considered intractable. Moreover, the patients can check the presence of TCH by themselves and prevent the recurrence of TMD. Therefore, the sense of incurability that "TMD is a chronic disease which relapses repeatedly" has been almost eliminated.

I have already published several textbooks concerning TCH correction training and rehabilitation training respectively. It is critical to proceed both training as two wheels of a bicycle in TMD treatment. The intent of this publication is to organize the treatment concept as "Kino method". Diagnosis of etiology and symptoms, as well as treatment tips are clearly explained to make this TMD treatment guide book literally practical.

As one of our new attempts, English explanation is basically written throghout the text. TCH correction training is a highly effective and non-invasive treatment, unfortunately, it is still unfamiliar overseas. Nevertheless, tremendous interest in mastering TCH correction training has been expressed by many visitors and foreign students from various parts of the world who are impressed by these excellent treatment options originated in Japan. In many regions, including Asian countries, many of the dental literatures are written in English. Appended English in this book will help foreign dentists understand our treatment concept, and clinically practice it in their home countries.

At the same time, the increase of tourists from overseas could give Japanese dentists opportunities to examine foreign patients with TMD. This book should be utilized as a chairside guide in such situations. Appendices of questionnaire forms are also provided with English versions, which are expected to help take care of foreign patients smoothly.

I'm hoping that utilization of this book by many dentists would globally innovate TMD treatment modalities to relieve all TMD patients of their symptoms.

June, 2019

Koji Kino

Contents

Chapter 1 木野メソッドの治療コンセプト　　木野 孔司　8
Treatment concept of Kino method　　Koji Kino

1. 顎関節症の病態と病因の両方にアプローチする
   An approach to both aspects of TMD: symptoms and causes
2. 木野メソッドが高い治療効果を得られる理由
   Reasons for high therapeutic effectiveness of Kino method

Chapter 2 顎関節症患者に対する精神医学的医療面接　　和気 裕之　12
Psychiatric medical interview for TMD patients　　Hiroyuki Wake

1. 医療面接の基本
   Basic principles of the medical interview
2. 顎関節症患者の特徴をふまえた精神医学的医療面接
   Psychiatric medical interview based on characteristics of TMD
3. 精神科への対診
   Judgment of consultation on psychiatry

Chapter 3 顎関節症の病態診断　　儀武 啓幸　20
Diagnosis of TMD based on pathological conditions　　Hiroyuki Yoshitake

1. 顎関節症の診断
   Diagnosis of TMD
2. 診察・検査のポイント
   Consultation and examination of TMD
3. 顎関節症の病態分類
   Classification of TMD by The Japanese Society for Temporomandibular Joint
4. 医歯大式病型分類
   Classification of TMD by Tokyo Medical and Dental University

Chapter 4 顎関節症の病態治療　　儀武 啓幸　30
Symptomatic treatment of TMD　　Hiroyuki Yoshitake

1. リハビリトレーニングの特徴と効果
   Features and effects of rehabilitation training
2. リハビリトレーニングの種類と適応症
   Types of rehabilitation training and their indications

Chapter 5 顎関節症の病因診断　　佐藤 文明　37
Etiological diagnosis of TMD　　Fumiaki Sato

1. 顎関節症の病因の考え方―単一病因説と多因子病因説―
   Interpretations of pathogenesis of TMD―Single etiology and multifactorial etiology―
2. どの寄与因子を顎関節症治療のターゲットとするか?
   Which contributing factors should be targeted for treatment of TMD?
3. TCHとは
   Tooth contacting habit
4. 顎関節症の寄与因子としてのTCH
   TCH as a contributing factor of TMD

5. TCHはどのように定着するのか？
How does TCH become established?

6. TCHの診察と診断
Examination and diagnosis of TCH

Chapter 6　顎関節症の病因治療　　　佐藤 文明　52
Etiological treatment of TMD　　　Fumiaki Sato

1. 顎関節症の病因治療の概念
Concept of etiological treatment of TMD

2. TCH是正訓練にあたっての注意点
Important points of TCH correction training

3. 習慣逆転法によるTCHの是正
Correction training of TCH by habit reversal method

4. TCH是正の評価
Evaluation of TCH correction

Chapter 7　治療終了時の患者指導と再発時の対応　　　木野 孔司　63
Patient guidance at the end of TMD treatment and management of recurrence　　　Koji Kino

1. 治療終了とする判断基準
Criteria for terminating TMD treatment

2. 再発防止のため患者に伝えておくべきこと
Essential information for patients to prevent recurrence

3. 補綴治療・インプラント治療・矯正歯科治療等の開始時期
Timing for initiation of prosthodontics, implant therapy and orthodontics

4. 顎関節症再発時の対応
How to manage relapsed TMD

Chapter 8　木野メソッドによる治療例　　　木野 孔司　70
Cases treated with Kino method　　　Koji Kino

Case 1　左咀嚼筋痛障害
Left myalgia of the masticatory muscle

Case 2　右顎関節円板障害・右咀嚼筋痛障害
Right TMJ disc derangement, right myalgia of the masticatory muscle

Case 3　かくれ顎関節症に咬合違和感を併発
Hidden-TMD accompanied by occlusal dysesthesia

Appendix　顎関節症初診時質問票，精神医学的面接質問票，生活・行動要因調査票
Questionnaire for New TMD Patient, Psychiatric Questionnaire, Questionnaire on Living/Behavioral Factors

---

本書では，海外の歯科医師にわれわれの治療コンセプトを紹介したいとの思いから，英文のサマリーを付し，図表にも英語を併記した．日本の歯科医師には，顎関節症で外国人患者が来院した際にチェアサイドで活用いただきたい．
Our hope to offer the treatment concept introduced in this book to many foreign dentists motivated us to install English summary for each chapter and translate figures/tables/questionnaire forms into English. Globally may this attempt help innovate TMD treatment modalities by practicing Kino method in their home countries.

Treatment concept of Kino method

木野メソッドの治療コンセプト

木野孔司 *Koji Kino*

顎関節症の病態と病因の両方にアプローチする
An approach to both aspects of TMD: symptoms and causes

　顎関節症の治療が難しいと言われるのはなぜだろうか？　臨床の現場で標準的に用いられる，鎮痛薬による薬物療法やスプリント治療を行っても，症状が完全に消失する患者が少なく，通院が長期化することが多いためであろう．

　どのような疾患の治療においても，病態と病因の双方に対するアプローチが必要であり，顎関節症治療も同様である．これまで行われてきた顎関節症の治療法では，どちらかへのアプローチが欠けていたために，治療の長期化を招いたと考えられる．

1) 顎関節症の病態に対する治療

　顎関節症の病態を改善するための治療としては，薬物療法以外に冷温罨法，マッサージ，電気療法，緩徐な開口訓練などが行われてきた．これらの治療でも多少の効果はみられるが，科学的治験に基づいて有効性が報告されているのは薬物療法のみである．

　本書で紹介する「リハビリトレーニング」は，東京医科歯科大学第一口腔外科で試行錯誤しながら行ってきた運動療法が基になっており，これまでの歯科臨床では行われたことのない，痛みを伴う積極的な訓練療法である．患者が自らの手指を用いて行うこの方法は，スプリント治療に比べ有意に効果が高いことが示されている[1]．

2) 顎関節症の病因に対する治療

　以前は，咬み合わせ不良が顎関節症の単一病因であると信じられ，顎関節症を改善するために咬合療法が行われていたが，治療効果は不確実であった．

　その後，咬合以外にも顎関節症の発症にかかわる因子が多く見つかり，上下歯列接触癖（Tooth Contacting Habit: TCH）が多くの顎関節症患者において最大の病因であることが明らかとなった[2]．したがって，TCHをもつ顎関節症患者に対しては，病因に対する治療としてTCHの是正を行うのが有効である．

　われわれは，長年にわたり顎関節症の研究と臨床に携わるなかで，自転車の両輪のように，病態に対してはリハビリトレーニングを，病因に対してはTCH是正訓練を並行して行うこと

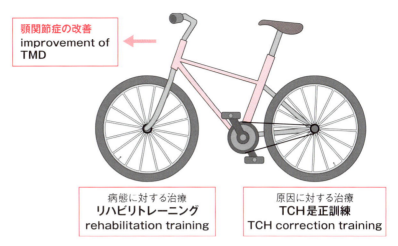

Fig. 1-1 木野メソッドによる顎関節症治療のコンセプト
自転車の両輪のように，病態に対してはリハビリトレーニングを，病因に対してはTCH是正訓練を並行して行うことで，確実な治療効果が得られる

Fig. 1-1 Two wheels of Kino method
Predictable therapeutic effects can be obtained by performing rehabilitation training for reducing symptoms and TCH correction training for eliminating etiology in parallel, like the two wheels of a bicycle.

により，確実な治療効果を得てきた（**Fig. 1-1**）．

本書では，その治療コンセプトに則って，診断と治療の実際を紹介していきたい．この木野メソッドを実施することで，これまでの顎関節症治療の効果を大きく越える治療結果が得られるはずである．

1. An approach to both aspects of TMD: symptoms and causes

Difficulties of temporomandibular disorder (TMD) treatment stem from the fact that complete remission of symptoms are rarely achieved by traditional modalities, such as pharmacotherapy or occlusal appliance therapy. An approach to causes and symptoms in parallel has become imperative for TMD patients.

1) Management of TMD symptoms

"Rehabilitation training" introduced in this text is based on exercise therapy that has been studied in The First Department of Oral and Maxillofacial Surgery, Tokyo Medical and Dental University. This patient-performed method is an aggressive, pain-evoked training. However, it is significantly more effective than oral appliance therapy[1].

2) Management of TMJ causes

Tooth Contacting Habit (TCH) is now affirmed to be a major etiology in a large number of TMD patients[2]. Therefore, from the perspective of etiological management, corrective measures for TCH are undoubtedly effective.

Management of symptoms and causes work closely together like the two wheels of a bicycle (**Fig. 1-1**), which results in positive treatment outcomes.

2 木野メソッドが高い治療効果を得られる理由
Reasons for high therapeutic effectiveness of Kino method

　顎関節症は，自然経過のよい疾患である[3]．安静を指示するだけで，徐々に症状が軽減する患者も少なくない．

　しかしながら，痛みや開口障害などの症状がなかなか改善しない場合には，生活への支障が大きいため，確実な治療結果が求められる．木野メソッドの両輪であるリハビリトレーニングとTCH是正訓練が高い治療効果を得られる理由を以下に示す．

1) リハビリトレーニングの特徴

　顎関節症の病態に対する治療として行うリハビリトレーニングは，「よく動く関節に痛みはない」という，整形外科領域においては経験則から常識となっている考え方を基本コンセプトとしている (**Fig. 1-2**)．

　顎関節症に病態が似ている膝関節症を考えていただきたい．膝関節症では，急性期には安静にすることもあるが，急性痛が治まったら理学療法士が積極的に膝を動かすトレーニングを開始する．関節は最大の可動域を維持することによって，関節周囲に血液を集め，そこからつくられた滑液で関節内部に栄養と酸素を供給している．そのため，関節の可動域が減少すると，関節腔内組織への栄養供給が低下し，周囲組織が破壊されて関節の変形を引き起こす．それとともに，周囲滑膜の神経終末を刺激する物質が産生され，痛みが生じる．痛みのためさらに関節を動かさずにいると，関節周辺組織への栄養供給がいっそう悪くなり，悪循環に拍車がかかってしまう．

　したがって，関節の変形や痛みがあっても，可動域を大きくすることで血液供給を増加させ，関節周辺の組織に栄養を与え，疼痛関連物質の産生を抑えることが重要である．痛みを訴えない人の膝関節は，変形していても可動域が大きいことが知られている．

　顎関節においても膝関節と同様，関節を動かすトレーニングを継続することで，可動域の増加と痛みの軽減が図れる．リハビリトレーニングの詳細は4章で述べるが，痛みを伴うことが特徴である．患者に痛みを与える手法をためらう歯科医もいるだろうが，リハビリトレーニングに伴う痛みは歯痛のように激烈なものではなく，トレーニングしているうちに慣れてくる．患者はしばしば「痛くて口を開けられません」と言うが，「口を開けないから痛いのです」と説明できるようになっていただきたい．リハビリトレーニングを成功させるには，「痛みを与えて楽にする」という発想の転換が必要である．

2) TCH是正訓練の特徴

　患者が顎関節症の最大病因であるTCHを有する場合は，6章に紹介する方法で是正を行う．患者みずから行動を変える（癖をやめる）ために，習慣逆転法という，チック症状や吃音の改善に効果が報告されている手法を用いる．ヒトが本来もっている「上下の歯が触れたら離す」という反射機構を再獲得させる訓練であるため，これまで反射を戻せなかった患者はおらず，100％再獲得できる．

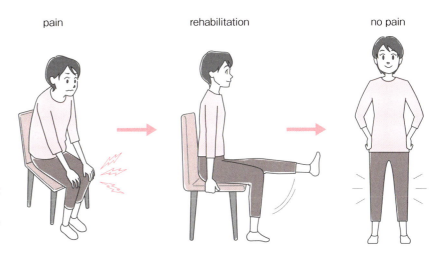

Fig. 1-2 リハビリトレーニングの基本となる考え方「よく動く関節に痛みはない」
Fig. 1-2 There is no pain in freely movable joints.

また，リハビリトレーニングもTCH是正訓練も，患者が自身で毎日行えることが大きな特徴である．歯科医院では最初に指導を行って，その後は定期的に確認し，必要に応じて改善を指示するだけでよく，特別な機器も必要ない．

2. Reasons for high therapeutic effectiveness of Kino method

In general, TMD follows a good natural course[3]. Some patients' symptoms improve merely with rest. However, in case of patients with prolonged symptoms, such as pain and limited mouth opening, their daily difficulties should be predictably treated. Rationales for rehabilitation training and TCH correction training, which constitute the two wheels of Kino method are explained below:

1) Rehabilitation training

"There is no pain in freely movable joints" (**Fig. 1-2**) is a common empirical rule in the field of orthopedic surgery, where the rehabilitation training stands on. This rule is also true for TMJ. Regardless of the existence of joint deformity or pain, continuing the exercise expands range of motion, increases blood supply, nourishes joint-surrounding tissues, inhibits pain-producing substances, and thus results in pain relief. As like cures like, pain cures pain.

2) TCH correction training

A behavioral modification to quit the habit called "habit reversal" method is applied to patients with TCH. This method is based on the congenital reflex that teeth separate as they contact with each other.

Patients can perform these training by themselves every day, without necessitating any special equipment.

References

1) Haketa T, Kino K, Sugisaki M, et al. Randomized clinical trial of treatment for TMJ disc displacement. *J Dent Res*. 2010; **89**: 1259-1263.
2) Sato F, Kino K, Sugisaki M, et al. Teeth contacting habit as a contributing factor to chronic pain in patients with temporomandibular disorders. *J Med Dent Sci*. 2006; **53**: 103-109.
3) Kurita K, Westesson PL, Yuasa H, et al. Natural course of untreated symptomatic temporomandibular joint disc displacement without reduction. *J Dent Res*. 1998; **77**: 361-365.

Chapter 2

Psychiatric medical interview for TMD patients

顎関節症患者に対する精神医学的医療面接

和気裕之 *Hiroyuki Wake*

1 医療面接の基本
Basic principles of the medical interview

顎関節症を正しく診断するには，医療面接（問診）・診察（視診・触診）・身体的検査が重要である．病態と病因にアプローチを行う木野メソッドにおいては，医療面接と身体的検査の結果に基づき，病態と病因に対する診断を行う．病態診断と病因診断はそれぞれ3章と5章で詳述し，本章では主に精神面への配慮が必要な顎関節症患者に対する精神医学的医療面接について述べる．

1) 医療面接の目的
医療面接の目的は，信頼関係の構築，医療情報の収集，そして患者教育と動機づけである（**Fig. 2-1**）．情報の収集に役立つ初診時質問票の書式は，巻末の付録No.1を参照されたい．

2) 医療面接の流れ
初めに，開放型の質問（答えを自由に選べる質問）を行う．例としては，「今日は，どのようなことでいらっしゃいましたか」「その症状は，いつ頃始まって，どうなったか詳しく教えてください」等である．次に，「その後はどうなりましたか」「それから？」等，話を促進させる中立型の質問を行う．後半は「食事はできますか」「よく眠れますか」等，「はい」または「いいえ」で答えを求める閉鎖型の質問を行い，診断や治療に役立つ情報を収集する（**Fig. 2-2**）．

患者の様子に応じて，「それは大変でしたね」「とてもつらかったですね」等の，共感的な言葉や態度を示すことも，ラポールの形成や治療をスムーズに進めるうえで大切である．

1. Basic principles of the medical interview

In Kino method, pathological conditions and causes are diagnosed from results of the medical interview and physical examination. Aims of the medical interview are listed in **Fig. 2-1**. The questionnaire for initial consultation represented in Appendix No.1 would be of help to collect patient information. Following the sequence as **Fig. 2-2** makes the medical interview go smoothly. When psychosocial considerations are required for certain patients, psychiatric medical interview should be applied.

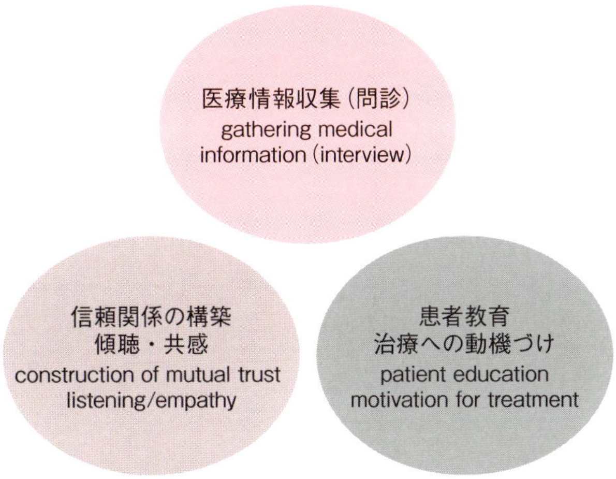

Fig. 2-1　医療面接の目的
Fig. 2-1　Aims of the medical interview

- 医療情報収集（問診） gathering medical information (interview)
- 信頼関係の構築 傾聴・共感 construction of mutual trust listening/empathy
- 患者教育 治療への動機づけ patient education motivation for treatment

開放型の質問 (open-ended questions)
答えを自由に選べる質問
「今日はどのようなことでいらっしゃいましたか？」
a question that cannot be answered with "yes" or "no"
e.g. "What brings you here today?"

中立型の質問 (neutral questions)
開放型や閉鎖型ではなく，話を促進させる質問
「その後はどうなりましたか？」
a question that encourage talking
e.g. "What has become of your problem after that?"

閉鎖型の質問 (closed-ended questions)
「はい」または「いいえ」で答える質問
「よく眠れますか？」
a question that can be answered with "yes" or "no"
e.g. "Do you sleep well at night?"

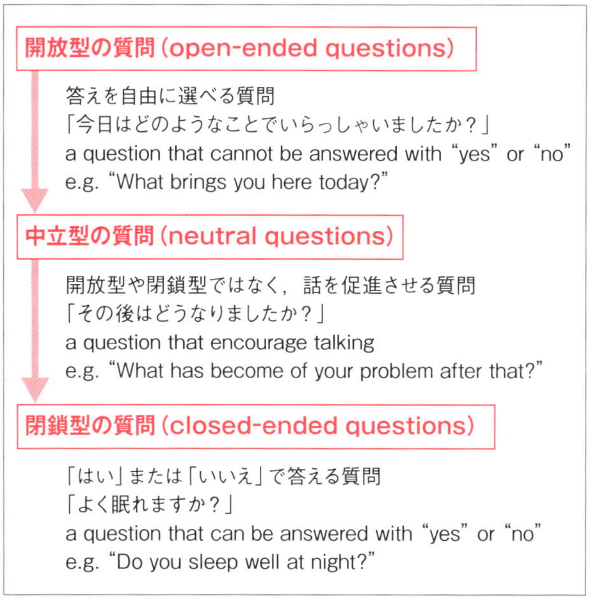

Fig. 2-2　医療面接の流れ
Fig. 2-2　Flow of the medical interview

2 顎関節症患者の特徴をふまえた精神医学的医療面接
Psychiatric medical interview based on characteristics of TMD

1) 精神医学的医療面接

　顎関節症は，患者の心理社会的要因が発症や経過に影響を及ぼすbio-psychosocial modelに当てはまる疾患であり，身体面と心理社会面の評価と対応が必要である．不安や抑うつ気分の亢進は全身の筋緊張を招き，TCHを是正しても治療効果が上がりにくいため，心理社会面に配慮が必要と思われる患者に対しては，精神医学的医療面接が有用である．

　精神医学的医療面接には，診断面接と治療面接の2つの側面がある．初診時（あるいは治療期間中）に精神的な問題が疑われた患者に対しては，巻末の付録No.2にあるような質問票を用いて精神医学的な評価を行い，後述するMW分類によって対応を決定する．また，顎関節症の治療における病態説明，生活習慣指導，セルフケア指導等は，対話の形をとることから精神医学的医療面接のなかで行っていく[1]．治療の詳細は4章と6章を参照していただきたい．

2) 精神医学的医療面接を行う必要がある患者の判断

　精神医学的医療面接が必要な患者の傾向をTab. 2-1に示す．

　付き添いの存在は，患者が何らかの問題により一人で診察を受けることが難しい状態を示す．問題には，会話が不自由等の身体的なもの以外に，認知症や精神疾患等がある．入室時の表情や様子，問診への受け答えから，認知症や抑うつ状態等が読み取れる場合もある．

　質問票の記載内容は，患者の事実の他に思考（解釈モデル）や感情を表している．言いにくいことは記載しないという場合もあれば，実際よりもよく見せたい，あるいは悪く見せたい等

Tab. 2-1　精神医学的医療面接が必要な患者の傾向

(1) 来院・入室時の状況	①患者に付き添いがいる ②患者に付き添いがおり，患者は一人で入室 ③患者と付き添いが一緒に入室
(2) 入室時の表情等	①うつむいている ②視線を合わせない ③挨拶をしない ④表情が暗い (笑顔がない) ⑤怒りの表情が現れている ⑥泣いている
(3) 問診への受け答え	①質問に答えない ②話が止まらない (多弁) ③質問とは異なる回答をする ④同じ話を繰り返し，まとまりがつかない (迂遠) ⑤質問にのみ答え，自らは話さない
(4) 資料の持参	①自分で作成した過去の治療記録 (文字，絵等) を持参する ②歯列模型やX線写真等を持参する
(5) 質問票の記載状況	①症状や経過を詳細に記載する ②記載に時間がかかる ③前医への不満や医療不信を記載する ④質問内容とは異なる回答をする

の心理が働くこともある．したがって，患者の前で質問票を読みながら，記載内容を確認することが重要である．また，自身の治療に関する資料を持参する行為は，過去の治療に対する不満や不信，医療者に自分の状態や気持ちを強く伝えたい等の表現であることが多い．

医療面接から得られる情報では，以下のようなものに注意する．

① **主訴**：多愁訴である．
② **現病歴**：経過が長い．同じ症状で複数の医療機関を受診している[2]．各種の検査で原因が見つからない．また，すでに受けた薬物療法やスプリント治療等の治療効果がない．慢性疼痛に該当する痛みがある．不定愁訴と考えられる身体症状を有する．
③ **既往歴**：うつ病等の精神疾患がある．また，内科等で自律神経失調症と診断されたり，向精神薬の投与を受けたりしたことがある．歯科では，舌痛症，口腔異常感症，口臭恐怖症，咬合感覚異常症 (いわゆる phantom bite syndrome) 等の歯科心身症の既往がある．
④ **家族歴**：遺伝的な負因がある．
⑤ **現症**：痛みの部位が多い．症状が移動する．
⑥ **日常の生活状況**：社会生活 (学校，職場，地域等) や，家族関係 (親子，夫婦，兄弟，パートナー等) に問題がある．日常生活の質 (QOL) の低下は，顎関節症の症状だけでなく，腰痛や生理痛等の身体症状，不眠や食欲の低下，疲労感，不安感・憂うつ感等の気分，気力や能率の低下等を尋ねることで把握できることが多い．

家族関係の問題は，家族歴を聴取するなかで問診すると患者は答えやすい．ストレスは，ストレッサーによる身体的・心理的・行動的な歪みを指すが，顎関節症患者では家族関係によるものが多い (**Fig. 2-3**)[3]．

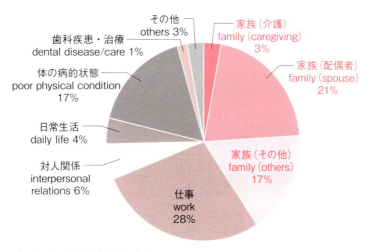

Fig.2-3 顎関節症患者の抱えるストレス
口腔外科のリエゾン外来で診療した顎関節症患者135名における調査結果(中久木ほか 2012より)[3]. 家族に関するものが約40%を占める(赤字部分)

Fig. 2-3 Stress found in TMD patients at Oral Surgery Section, Liaison Clinic (135 cases)

2. Psychiatric medical interview based on characteristics of TMD

As temporomandibular disorder (TMD) should be comprehended from the perspective of biopsychosocial model, evaluation and management of physical and psychosocial aspects are necessary.

Because psychiatric medical interview has two roles, one is diagnosis and the other is treatment, it is useful for interviewing TMD patients. The questionnaire shown in Appendix No.2 is suitable for this kind of interview.

Tendencies of patients to whom psychiatric medical interview is applied are as follows.

・Attendants are with them. They come into the office with dark expression, no eye contact, no greeting, anger, or tears. During the interview, they give no reply or unrelated answers to questions, keep talking or repeating the same story, etc.

・Questionnaire statements: detailed descriptions of symptoms and progress, dissatisfaction with the previous dentist, medical distrust, and unrelated answers to the questions. Some patients bring their original therapy records (written, drawn, or others), dental casts and X-rays from previous dentists.

・Medical interview: they accompany more than one symptoms, current medical histories with prolonged progress, a symptom consulted at different medical care providers, no etiology identified by various examinations, ineffectiveness of past treatment such as pharmacotherapy or oral appliance therapy, chronic pain, and physical symptoms assumed to be unidentified complaints syndrome.

・Past history: mental disorders such as depression, diagnosis of autonomic imbalance, psychotropic administration, dental psychosomatic disorders such as glossalgia, oral dysesthesia, halitophobia, occlusal dysesthesia (so-called phantom bite syndrome)

・Family history: genetic negative factors

・Present condition: multiple pains, migration of symptoms

・Living conditions: difficulties of social life in schools, workplaces, communities, etc., problems in family relationship with parents, siblings, spouses, partners (**Fig. 2-3**), etc.

3 精神科への対診
Judgment of consultation on psychiatry

　精神科に対診を求める患者の判定は，前述の精神医学的医療面接や心理検査，また治療経過から行う．歯科医師は精神疾患を診断する必要はないが，精神医学的な問題を有する患者を評価して，治療方針を誤らないことが重要である．ここでは，筆者が開発に携わった簡便な患者の分類法（MW分類；宮岡・和気 2001）[4-6]と，そのタイプ別の対応法を述べる．

1) 心身医学・精神医学的な対応を要する患者の分類（MW分類）と対応法

　MW分類ではまず，精神医学的医療面接と身体的検査の結果から，自覚症状と他覚所見の関係を検討する．そして，自覚症状を説明できる他覚所見が認められない患者をType A，他覚所見は認められるものの，それが自覚症状を十分に説明できるものではない患者をType B，他覚所見があり，同時に統合失調症のような明らかな精神疾患がある患者をType C，症状の発症や経過にストレスが密接に関係している患者をType Dとする（**Fig. 2-4**）[7]．

① Type A：自覚症状タイプ

　【例】顎関節部と咬筋部に自発痛と開口時痛がある．痛みは激痛で触診ができない．開口量は一横指．その他に食欲低下，不眠がある．患者は休職しており，日常生活のレベルは著しく低下している．顎顔面部の画像検査では異常がなく，炎症や腫瘍等を疑う所見もない．

　【病態】患者が自覚症状を訴えているにもかかわらず，詳細な診察や検査の結果，歯科および医科の身体疾患の可能性が否定される場合は，身体表現性障害や抑うつ障害群，不安障害群に含まれる精神疾患の身体化症状の可能性が考えられる．身体化にはさまざまな解釈があるが，ここでは「不安や心理社会的ストレスを身体症状として訴えること」として用いる．

　【対応】まず，歯科的な所見が見つからなくても焦らないことである．侵襲的な検査や診断的な治療は慎重に行う．さらに，経過を診て精神科等との連携や紹介を行う．

② Type B：自覚症状・他覚所見乖離タイプ

　【例】顎関節部に圧痛と開口時痛がある．その他に，咬合異常感，頭痛，耳閉感，後頸部・肩部の痛みと痺れ感がある．開口量は二横指半．開口時に顎関節雑音（クリック）を触知する．顎顔面部の画像検査では異常がないが，不正咬合がある．脳神経外科，耳鼻咽喉科の検査で異常がない．

　【病態】診察や検査で他覚所見は見つかるが，自覚症状がその所見に起因していると断定できない．

　【対応】所見を見つけても安心せず，不可逆的な処置は控えて，所見の説明や可逆的な治療で経過を診る．診断的治療を行う場合は，症状が改善・不変・悪化する可能性があること，また治療をしなかった場合のメリットとデメリットを説明して患者の同意を得る．不可逆的な治療を行う場合は，承諾書を作成する．

　なお，Type AとBは，身体疾患を発見できていない可能性もあるため，経過を診て再検査を行う．

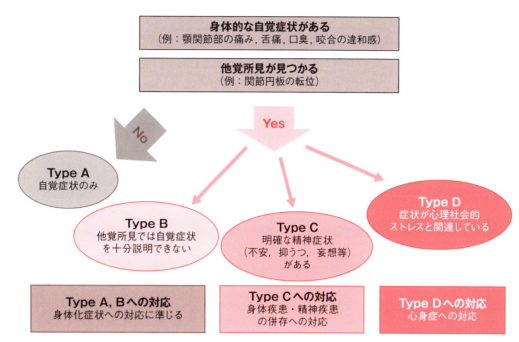

Fig. 2-4 MW分類
心身医学・精神医学的な対応を要する患者の分類（宮岡・和気 2001）と，タイプ別対応のフローチャート（和気 2015より）[7]

③ Type C：身体疾患・精神疾患併存タイプ

【例】顎関節部の開口時痛がある．開口時に顎関節雑音（クリック）があり，時々顎が引っかかって開かなくなる．画像検査では下顎頭の変形が認められる．不安障害で精神科に通院し，薬物療法を受けている．家族との関係から精神的に不安定になると，顎の痛みがつらくなる．

【病態】明確な身体疾患が存在し，かつ明らかな不安や抑うつ，妄想等が認められる場合や，精神疾患で治療を受けている．

【対応】原則的には顎関節症と精神疾患の治療を同時に行うが，緊急性のあるほうを優先する．両方の疾患の相互関係や薬物の併用禁忌に注意する．

通院中の精神科等がある場合は，歯科治療の可否を問い合わせる．精神科や心療内科へ紹介する場合は，歯科でも併診することを患者に約束する．

④ Type D：心身症タイプ

【例】咬筋部と側頭筋部に開口時痛と圧痛がある．開口量は三横指．画像検査は異常なし．職場の環境で悩んでおり，仕事量が多い時や人間関係が悪い時に痛みが悪化する．顕著な抑うつ症状は認めない．

【病態】明らかな身体疾患があり，その症状がストレスによって発症したり，悪化したりする．Type A〜Cには該当しない．

【対応】歯科での心身医学療法等が中心となるが，顎関節症の治療（リハビリトレーニングとTCH是正訓練）も行う．ただし，ほとんどの精神疾患はストレスの影響を受けることから，安易に心身症と判断すべきではない．なお，患者の有するストレスが深刻な場合は，精神科や心療内科へ紹介する．

1. 診察と検査の結果から，症状の原因となる歯科疾患は見つからなかったことを伝える
2. 同様の症状は医科の疾患でも現れる場合があることを説明し，医科の診察を提案する
3. 不眠や不安感，憂うつ感等があれば，その問題を取り上げて精神科や心療内科の専門医に相談することを提案する
4. 精神科や心療内科は，検査で異常の見つからない身体の慢性的な痛みや違和感を専門に扱っていることを説明する
5. 歯科では，精神科や心療内科へ紹介後も診察を行うことを約束する．また，必要に応じて検査を行う
6. 十分な説明を行っても理解が得られない場合は，家族の来院を促し，上記と同様の説明を行って協力を得る

Fig. 2-5 精神科や心療内科へ患者を紹介する時のポイント

2) 精神科との医療連携

上記に示した患者の治療では，精神科との医療連携が必要となる場合が多い．患者を精神科に紹介する際のポイントは，「自分の専門外のことを専門医に依頼するが，その後も自覚症状のある顎や口については継続して診ていく」ことを患者にしっかり伝えることである．これにより，患者は歯科医師から見捨てられたと受け取らず，精神科への通院も続くことが多い．また，理解力・判断力・記憶力等の問題から紹介が困難と考えられた場合は，家族等の協力を得る[7]（**Fig. 2-5**）．

3. Judgment of consultation on psychiatry

The necessity of consultation on psychiatry is determined on the base of above mentioned psychiatric medical interview, psychological examination, and treatment progress. Dental physicians are not necessary to diagnose mental disorders, but evaluation of patients with psychiatric problems is important to select appropriate treatment courses.

A convenient method to classify patients into four categories after psychiatric medical interview and physical examinations, called MW classification (**Fig. 2-4**), and each management procedure for these classified patients are described below.

1) **Classification of patients who need psychosomatic and psychiatric management**

Initially, the relationship of subjective symptoms and objective findings are assessed. A patient whose subjective symptoms are explainable by her/his objective findings is classified as Type A. A patient with objective findings which cannot fully describe her/his subjective symptoms is classified as Type B. A patient with objective findings who suffer from obvious mental disorder such as schizophrenia is classified as Type C. A patient whose stress is closely related to the onset and course of her/his symptoms is classified as Type D.

For Type A, dentists have no need to get confused with no findings. Care must be taken if invasive examination and diagnostic treatment are applied. Depending on the progress, cooperation with or referral to a psychiatrist is needed.

For Type B, the findings do not indicate irreversible interventions. Observation of progress and reversible treatment are recommended. If diagnostic treatment is needed, inform the possibility of getting better/no change/getting worse and obtain consent. In these types, reexamination may be required for possibly overlooked physical disorders.

For Type C, dental and psychiatric treatment are often provided in parallel, but urgency

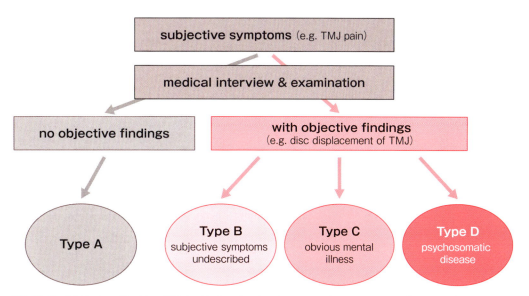

Fig. 2-4 MW classification (Wake H. Psychodentistry, psychosomatic medicine and psychiatic medicine for the dentist. Suna shobou, 2015.)[7]

can be prioritized. Enough understanding of interaction between both disorders and incompatible drugs is imperative. In case the patient has a psychiatrist, feasibility of dental treatment should be inquired. When the patient is referred to a psychiatrist, it is necessary to remind her/him that dental treatment continues along with psychiatric practice.

For Type D, psychosomatic therapy is mainly offered accompanying treatments for organic diseases. Patients with serious stress should be referred to psychiatry or psychosomatic medicine.

2) Cooperation with psychiatry

When a patient is referred to psychiatry, convince her/him that consultation on the psychiatric specialty is the prime purpose and subjective symptoms of jaw and mouth are continuously addressed in dental office. This contributes to avoiding the misunderstanding of patients to be forsaken by dentists, which helps them to keep attending psychiatric services. If comprehension, judgment and memory problems hinder the referral, family cooperation should be requested.

References

1) 澁谷智明, 和気裕之ほか. TMD患者（周辺群）への医療面接. ザ・クインテッセンス別冊/TMD YEARBOOK 2014 アゴの痛みに対処する—世界標準の新しいTMD診断基準「DC/TMD」の全貌—. クインテッセンス出版, 2014；66-70.
2) Miyachi H, Wake H, et al. Detecting mental disorders in dental patients with occlusion-related problems. *Psychiatry Clin Neurosci.* 2007; **61**(3): 313-319.
3) 中久木康一, 和気裕之ほか. 口腔外科における精神科リエゾン診療外来を10年間に受診した患者の臨床統計的検討. 日歯心身. 2013；**27**（1・2）：10-18.
4) 和気裕之. 顎関節症患者に対する心身医学的なアプローチ. 顎頭蓋誌. 2001；**14**（1）：1-13.
5) 和気裕之, 小見山 道. 顎関節症患者の心身医学的な治療の変遷. 補綴誌. 2012；**4**（3）：256-266.
6) 和気裕之, 小見山 道. 顎関節症診療における歯科医師と精神科医の連携. 日顎誌. 2014；**26**（3）：183-190.
7) 和気裕之. サイコ・デンティストリー 歯科医のための心身医学・精神医学 第2版. 砂書房, 2015；153.

Chapter 3

Diagnosis of TMD based on pathological conditions

顎関節症の病態診断

儀武啓幸 *Hiroyuki Yoshitake*

顎関節症の診断
Diagnosis of TMD

　木野メソッドの顎関節症治療では，顎関節症の病態と病因双方に対しアプローチを行うが，本章では病態の診断について述べていく．医療面接と身体的検査の結果を基に，問題のある身体部位（顎関節なのか，咀嚼筋なのか，その双方であるのか）とその病態の診断を行い，リハビリトレーニングによる治療の適応か否かを判断する．

1) 顎関節症の概念

　まず，顎関節症とはどのような疾患であるのか，きちんと理解しておく必要がある．日本顎関節学会による顎関節症の概念(2013年)では，「顎関節症は，顎関節や咀嚼筋の疼痛，関節（雑）音，開口障害あるいは顎運動異常を主要症候とする障害の包括的診断名である．その病態は咀嚼筋痛障害，顎関節痛障害，顎関節円板障害および変形性顎関節症である」とされている[1]．

2) 顎関節症の診断基準と鑑別診断

　「顎関節や咀嚼筋に症状がある」イコール「顎関節症」とはかぎらない．上記の顎関節症の概念にある主要徴候を1つ以上有することが確認でき，類似の症候を呈する疾患が除外されてはじめて顎関節症と診断することができる．

　顎関節症の痛みは機能時痛，すなわち開口時や閉口時，咀嚼時等に生じる顎関節部や咀嚼筋の痛みであり，基本的には患部の腫脹，発赤を生じることはない．実際には顎関節部に症状を有する患者の大部分は顎関節症であるが，顎関節症と類似した臨床症状を呈する疾患は多岐にわたるため，**Fig.3-1**に挙げた条件に該当する場合は顎関節症以外の疾患の可能性を考える必要がある（鑑別診断）．

3) かくれ顎関節症に注意！

　顎関節症に対して治療が行われた結果，症状の改善を認めたが寛解に至らないまま治療が中断し，放置されている症例が少なくない．顎関節症の症状が日常生活に支障をきたさない程度に残存し，ストレスやちょっとしたきっかけで症状が再燃してしまうこともある．そのような状態の患者群をわれわれは「かくれ顎関節症」と呼んでおり，留意する必要がある．

1. 開口障害25mm未満	1. maximum opening distance＜25mm
2. 2週間の一般的顎関節治療に反応しない，または悪化する	2. no response or worsening after common TMD treatments of 2 week
3. 顎関節部や咀嚼筋部の腫脹を認める	3. swelling of TMJ or masticatory muscles
4. 神経脱落症状を認める	4. neurological deficit
5. 発熱を伴う	5. fever
6. 他関節に症状を伴う	6. symptoms in other joints
7. 安静時痛を伴う	7. pain at rest

Fig. 3-1 顎関節症の鑑別診断のポイント（日本顎関節学会）[2]
Fig. 3-1 Differential diagnosis: signs and symptoms that rule out TMD (The Japanese Society for Temporomandibular Joint)

1. Diagnosis of TMD

TMD treatment using Kino method approaches symptoms and causes in parallel. In this chapter, diagnosis of pathological conditions is explained.

1) Definition of TMD

Temporomandibular disorder (TMD) is defined as a comprehensive diagnosis of disorders including i) pain of TMJ or masticatory muscles, ii) TMJ noises (clicking or crepitus), iii) limited mouth opening or limitation of mandibular movements. Pathological conditions of TMD contain myalgia of the masticatory muscle, arthralgia of TMJ, disc derangement, and osteoarthrosis/osteoarthritis.

2) Diagnostic criteria and differential diagnosis of TMD

Diagnosis of TMD requires involvement of one or more above mentioned conditions and elimination of diseases that exhibit similar symptoms. In case patients have any symptom shown in **Fig. 3-1**, TMD would be ruled out.

3) Hidden-temporomandibular disorder

Not a few TMD patients have been left without complete remission. Their symptoms could relapse easily by a small trigger like stress. Many of these patients with so-called hidden-temporomandibular disorder are unaware of TMD symptoms uncured.

2 診察・検査のポイント
Consultation and examination of TMD

顎関節症を正しく診断し，病態分類を行うには，厳密にはMRI等の高度な画像検査が必要だが，日常臨床で行うのは現実的ではない．そのような高度な検査を行わなくとも，適切な診察・検査と病歴聴取を行い，それらを評価することで顎関節症の治療に必要な病態診断を行うことは可能である．

1) 問診のポイント

病態を正しく把握するために，問診では「困っている症状は何か」「いつからなのか」「今までにどのように変化してきたのか」について確認する．巻末の付録No.1の初診時質問票に沿って話を進めていくとよい．

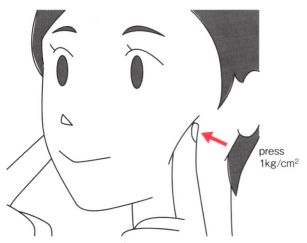

Fig. 3-2 痛みの部位の触診
診察する部位に両手の示指の腹を同時に当て，約1kg/cm²で圧迫する

Fig. 3-2 Palpation at sights of pain using finger pads

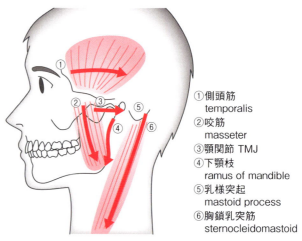

①側頭筋 temporalis
②咬筋 masseter
③顎関節 TMJ
④下顎枝 ramus of mandible
⑤乳様突起 mastoid process
⑥胸鎖乳突筋 sternocleidomastoid

Fig. 3-3 触診の順序
①〜⑥の順で，矢印方向に押していく．ただし，強い痛みを訴えている部位は後にする（木野 2015 より）[3]

Fig. 3-3 Sequence of palpation

2) 触診のポイント

痛みの部位の触診は示指の腹で両側から圧迫するように行い（**Fig. 3-2**），**Fig. 3-3**の順序で進める．

【咀嚼筋の触診のポイント】

下顎がどのような動きをした時に，どの筋が痛いのか？

➡ 手指によるポイントを押さえた触診で，どの部位に圧痛が生じるのかを的確に探し出していく．

【顎関節部の触診のポイント】

圧痛，開口時痛，咬合時痛，顎関節雑音は，それぞれ顎関節のどの部位において下顎がどう動いた時にどのように生じるのか？

➡ 顎関節症における顎関節痛は運動時痛（開口時，閉口時，側方運動時，前方運動時，咬合時，咀嚼時等に生じる痛み）である．どのような運動時にどこが痛いのかを手指による触診で入念に確かめる．

3) 開口障害の検査のポイント

開口量と，開閉口路の偏位，下顎の前方・側方運動時の滑走量を記録する．これらは，治療効果を評価する際の指標にもなる．

【開口量測定のポイント】

開口量は無痛・有痛・強制を区別して評価することが重要である（**Fig. 3-4**）．

無痛開口量：自分の力で開口し，顎関節や咀嚼筋に痛みを感じない範囲での最大開口のこと．徐々に開口してもらい，痛みを感じた時点で患者に手を挙げる等の合図をしてもらうと測定しやすい．成人男性における正常な開口量の目安は，無痛自力開口にて上下切歯間距離が40mm以上．

Chapter 3 顎関節症の病態診断

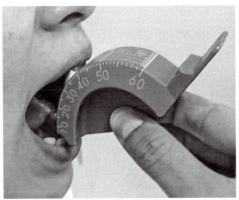
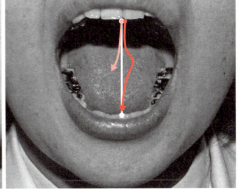

Fig. 3-4 開口量の測定と開閉口路の確認 (木野 2017より)[4]
成人男性の開口量の目安は40mm以上．開口路の偏位は，偏位した側の顎関節の可動域が制限されていることを示している

Fig. 3-4 Measurement of jaw-opening range (left) and identification of jaw opening and closing pathway (right)

　有痛開口量：自分の力で開口し，なおかつ痛みをこらえて開けられる最大の開口量のこと．

　強制開口量：自力開口ではなく，術者が介助して強制的に開口させた場合の最大開口量のこと．顎関節の物理的な可動範囲の限界を見極める意味がある．

　開閉口路の偏位：開口時に下顎が左右のどちら側に偏位するのかを観察する．もし右側に偏位するようであれば，右側の顎関節の可動域が制限されていることが示唆される．

2. Consultation and examination of TMD

1) Medical interview

The following points should be confirmed in medical interview, i) symptoms that the patient suffers from, ii) onset and course of them (see Appendix No. 1).

2) Palpation

Palpate sites of pain according to the methods shown in **Fig. 3-2** and **Fig. 3-3**.

Masticatory muscles: identify the muscle with pain in response to mandibular movements.

TMJ: identify components of TMJ where the pain localizes in response to mandibular movements.

3) Evaluation of mouth-opening

Maximal mouth-opening without pain: Interincisal distance is measured. This can be used as a base line of treatment. Normal value of adult male is 40 mm or more.

Maximal mouth-opening with pain: This refers to unassisted opening against pain of which site should be identified.

Assisted mouth-opening: This reflects physical border movement of TMJ.

Path of jaw opening and closing movements: Observe whether the deviation of the pathway exists (**Fig. 3-4**).

3 顎関節症の病態分類
Classification of TMD by The Japanese Society for Temporomandibular Joint

日本顎関節学会では，顎関節症をその病態から，咀嚼筋痛障害（Ⅰ型），顎関節痛障害（Ⅱ型），顎関節円板障害（Ⅲ型），および変形性顎関節症（Ⅳ型）の4つに分類している（**Fig. 3-5**，**Tab. 3-1**）．

1) 咀嚼筋痛障害（Ⅰ型）

下顎運動時，機能運動時，非機能運動時に惹起される咀嚼筋の痛みに関連する障害である[1]（**Fig. 3-6**）．これらの筋肉の運動時痛は筋の触診時あるいは最大開口時に認められ，その病態としては筋・筋膜痛が考えられているが，詳細な病態に関してはいまだに不明な点が多い．

2) 顎関節痛障害（Ⅱ型）

下顎運動時，機能運動時，非機能運動時に惹起される顎関節の痛みに関連する障害で[1]，外来性の外傷（顎顔面部の強打等）や内在性の外傷（過大開口，ブラキシズム等）によって生じる顎関節痛とそれによる運動障害を呈する状態である．滑膜，関節円板後部組織，関節包，関節靱帯の炎症や損傷により顎関節痛を生じる．

本病態が単独で発症することもあるが，顎関節円板障害（Ⅲ型）や変形性顎関節症（Ⅳ型）と併発することも多い．

3) 顎関節円板障害（Ⅲ型）

顎関節円板障害は，下顎頭-関節円板複合体を含むバイオメカニカルな関節内障害と定義される（顎関節内障と同義）[1]．

咀嚼筋痛障害（Ⅰ型）	myalgia of the masticatory muscle (type Ⅰ)
顎関節痛障害（Ⅱ型）	arthralgia of the temporomandibular joint (type Ⅱ)
顎関節円板障害（Ⅲ型）	temporomandibular joint disc derangement (type Ⅲ)
a：復位性	a：with reduction
b：非復位性	b：without reduction
変形性顎関節症（Ⅳ型）	osteoarthrosis/osteoarthritis of the temporomandibular joint (type Ⅳ)

註1：重複診断を認める
註2：顎関節円板障害には，関節円板内方転位，外方転位，後方転位，開口時の関節円板後方転位等を含む
註3：間欠ロックは，復位性顎関節円板障害に含める
Note 1: Multiple diagnosis permitted.
Note 2: TMJ disc derangement contains lateral displacement, posterior displacement, posterior displacement with jaw opening, etc.
Note 3: Intermittent lock resides in disc derangement with reduction.

Fig. 3-5 顎関節症の病態分類（日本顎関節学会 2013年）（日本顎関節学会 2018より作成）[1]
Fig. 3-5 Classification of TMD (Jpn Soc TMJ, 2013)

Tab. 3-1 顎関節症の各病態の特徴
Tab. 3-1 Features of each TMD condition

病態分類　pathological condition	臨床症状　clinical symptoms	病変部位　lesion sites
咀嚼筋痛障害（I型） myalgia of the masticatory muscle (type I)	運動時筋痛　muscle pain on motion 運動障害　motion disturbance	咬筋　masseter 側頭筋　temporalis 顎二腹筋　digastric 胸鎖乳突筋　sternocleidomastoid
顎関節痛障害（II型） arthralgia of the temporomandibular joint (type II)	運動時関節痛　joint pain on motion	顎関節部　TMJ
顎関節円板障害　復位性（IIIa型） temporomandibular joint disc derangement: with reduction (type IIIa)	開口時の顎関節雑音（クリック） 　TMJ noise with jaw opening 開閉口時の顎関節雑音（相反性クリック） 　TMJ noise with jaw opening/closing (reciprocal click) 運動時関節痛　joint pain on motion	関節円板　disc 滑膜　synovial membrane
顎関節円板障害　非復位性（IIIb型） temporomandibular joint disc derangement: without reduction (type IIIb)	顎関節雑音（クリック）の既往 　history of TMJ noise (click) 開口障害（クローズドロック） 　trismus (closed lock) 運動時関節痛　joint pain on motion	関節円板　disc 滑膜　synovial membrane
変形性顎関節症（IV型） osteoarthrosis/osteoarthritis of the temporomandibular joint (type IV)	顎関節雑音（特にクレピタス） 　TMJ noise (crepitus) 運動時関節痛　joint pain on motion	関節軟骨　articular cartilage 関節円板　disc 滑膜　synovial membrane 下顎頭　head of mandible 下顎窩　mandibular fossa

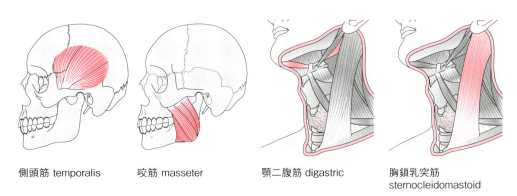

　　側頭筋 temporalis　　　咬筋 masseter　　　顎二腹筋 digastric　　　胸鎖乳突筋 sternocleidomastoid

Fig. 3-6　咀嚼筋痛障害を生じる部位（木野 2017を改変）[4]
Fig. 3-6　Sites of myalgia of the masticatory muscles

　多くの場合，関節円板は前方転位を呈しているが，後方転位や内外側への転位をきたすこともある．開口時に関節円板が下顎頭の上方に復位するか否かで，a型とb型に分類される（**Fig. 3-7**）．復位性関節円板前方転位では，開口時の関節円板の復位に伴い生じる顎関節雑音（クリック）が特徴的な臨床所見である．開口時に関節円板が復位しない場合は，クローズドロックの状態を呈する．

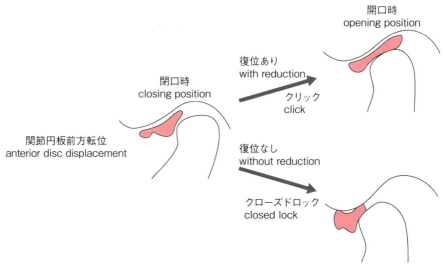

Fig. 3-7 顎関節円板障害
Fig. 3-7 Disc derangement of the temporomandibular joint

4) 変形性顎関節症（Ⅳ型）

　変形性顎関節症は，下顎頭と関節隆起の骨変化を伴う関節組織の破壊を特徴とする退行性変化と定義される[1]．特徴的な臨床症状は関節雑音（特にクレピタス：捻髪音）である．

3. Classification of TMD by The Japanese Society for Temporomandibular Joint（**Fig. 3-5**, **Tab. 3-1**）

1) Myalgia of the masticatory muscle（**Fig. 3-6**）
2) Arthralgia of the temporomandibular joint
3) Temporomandibular joint disc derangement（**Fig. 3-7**）
　　a: Anterior disc displacement with reduction
　　b: Anterior disc displacement without reduction
4) Osteoarthrosis/osteoarthritis of the temporomandibular joint

4 医歯大式病型分類
Classification of TMD by Tokyo Medical and Dental University

　　前述した日本顎関節学会の病態分類や国際的な顎関節症の診断分類であるDC/TMDは，診断が治療方針に直結していない．そこで，治療方針と連携した診断方法として木野が考案したのが「医歯大式病型分類」である（**Tab. 3-2**）．
　　診断は，**Fig. 3-8**のフローチャートに従うとスムーズに進めることができる．以下に，診断の流れを簡単に説明する．

Tab. 3-2 医歯大式病型分類
Tab. 3-2 Classification of TMD by TMDU (Tokyo Medical and Dental University)

病態 pathological condition	分類基準 classification criteria	医歯大式病型分類 TMDU classification	日本顎関節学会分類 classification by Jpn Soc TMJ
咀嚼筋痛障害 myalgia of the masticatory muscle	咀嚼筋痛単独 myalgia only	M M	I型 type I
	咀嚼筋痛＋顎関節痛 myalgia + arthralgia	MA MA	I型＋II型 type I + II
顎関節痛障害 arthralgia of the temporomandibular joint	顎関節痛単独 arthralgia only	A A	II型 type II
	顎関節痛＋咀嚼筋痛 arthralgia + myalgia	AM AM	II型＋I型 type II + I
顎関節雑音（クリック） TMJ noise (click)	クリックのみ（2週間未満） click only (<2 weeks)	CE CE	IIIa型 type IIIa
	クリックのみ（2週間以上） click only (≥2 weeks)	CO CO	IIIa型 type IIIa
	クリック時に痛みを伴う click + pain	CP CP	IIIa型＋II型 type IIIa + II
関節円板障害による開閉口障害 jaw opening/closing disturbance by TMJ disc derangement	クローズドロック（2週間未満） closed lock (<2 weeks)	LE LE	IIIb型（＋II型） type IIIb(+II)
	クローズドロック（2週間以上） closed lock (≥2 weeks)	LC LC	IIIb型（＋II型） type IIIb(+II)
	間欠性クローズドロック intermittent closed lock	IL IL	IIIb型（＋II型） type IIIb(+II)

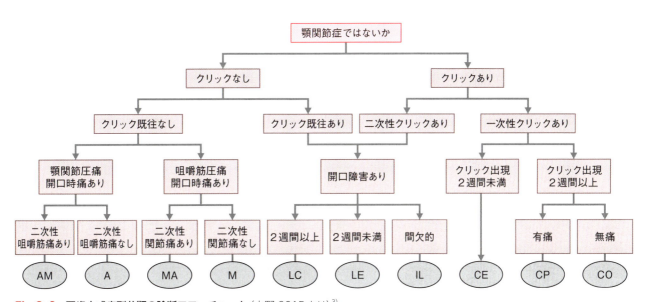

Fig. 3-8 医歯大式病型分類の診断フローチャート（木野 2015より）[3]

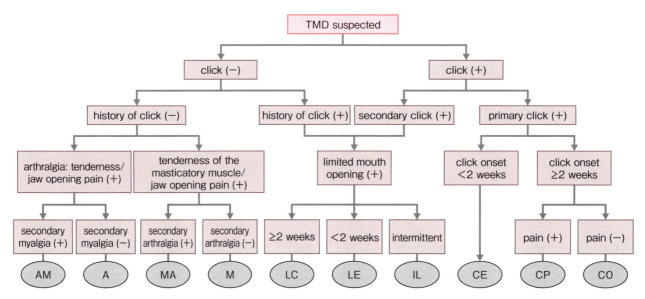

Fig. 3-8 Flowchart of classification of TMD developed by TMDU

Step 1
臨床症状と検査所見から顎関節症を疑ったら，まずはクリックの有無を確認する．

クリックあり → Step 4へ

クリックなし → Step 2，3へ

Step 2
Step 1でクリックを認めない症例において，過去にクリックの自覚があったか否か（クリック既往の有無）を問診により再度確認する．

Step 3
クリック既往なし → 顎関節痛（圧痛または開口時痛）の有無を確認

クリック既往あり → 開口障害の有無を確認

開口障害あり → 開口障害の期間を評価

Step 4
二次性クリックあり → Step 3へ

一次性クリックあり → クリックの期間を評価

クリックが2週間以上続いている場合 → 痛みの有無を評価

上記のStep 1〜4の手順を踏むことで，診断が絞られていく．4章で詳述するが，診断した病型によって治療方針を決定し，治療を進める．

なお，図中の二次性の痛みやクリックの病態は以下に述べるとおりである．

二次性咀嚼筋痛：初発の病態が顎関節痛である顎関節症において，顎関節痛が契機となり咀嚼筋の緊張が持続することによって筋の圧痛や開口時痛を生じるようになったと考えられる病態．

二次性顎関節痛：初発の病態が咀嚼筋痛である顎関節症において，咀嚼筋痛の持続的な緊張で顎関節の負荷が増大することにより顎関節部の圧痛や運動時痛を生じたと考えられる病態．

二次性クリック：非復位性関節円板前方転位において，その慢性期あるいは晩期に円板実質部が前方に位置するようになり下顎頭の前方滑走量が大きくなった症例において，円板下面の凹凸に下顎頭上面が引っかかり外れることで出現する小さなクリックのこと．患者の問診で「初めにしていたような大きな音とは違う」という回答があれば，円板転位初期の一次性クリックと区別できる．

4. Classification of TMD by Tokyo Medical and Dental University

In the classification by The Japanese Society for TMJ and DC/TMD, each diagnosis does not link to treatment methodology. This, then, has led Kino to develop a new classification of TMD that links directly to treatment strategy, described in **Tab. 3-2**.

Diagnosis would smoothly converge as proceeding with steps shown in **Fig. 3-8**.

Secondary symptoms described in this flowchart are defined as follows.

Secondary myalgia: A supposed condition in which incipient arthralgia that sustain tension of masticatory muscles triggers tenderness or jaw opening pain.

Secondary arthralgia: A supposed condition in which incipient myalgia that put an enhanced load on TMJ caused by persistent tension of masticatory muscles triggers tenderness or pain-on-motion of TMJ.

Secondary click: slight click produced when upper surface of condyle is caught and removed at the rugged lower surface of disc in chronic or late case that disc lies forward and condyle slides longer.

References

1) 日本顎関節学会 編. 新編 顎関節症 改訂版. 永末書店, 2018.
2) 日本顎関節学会. 顎関節症患者のための初期治療ガイドライン. http://kokuhoken.net/jstmj/publication/guideline.html
3) 木野孔司 編著. TCHのコントロールで治す顎関節症 第2版. 医歯薬出版, 2015.
4) 木野孔司 編著. 顎関節症のリハビリトレーニング. 医歯薬出版, 2017.

Chapter 4

Symptomatic treatment of TMD

顎関節症の病態治療

儀武啓幸 *Hiroyuki Yoshitake*

リハビリトレーニングの特徴と効果
Features and effects of rehabilitation training

　本章では顎関節症の病態に対する治療として，リハビリトレーニングと称する運動療法を紹介していく．リハビリトレーニングは，患者自身が院外で実施できる簡便な開口訓練である．高い治療効果が期待できるだけではなく，不可逆的な侵襲を加えることがないため，医療トラブルを避けることができるのも利点である．

　リハビリトレーニングの効果としては，繰り返しの運動による関節や靭帯，筋の痛みの閾値の上昇と関節構成体の適切なリモデリング，顎関節ではいわゆる関節ポンプの効果による関節腔内の炎症性物質や発痛物質の排出，咀嚼筋では血流の改善がもたらされると考えられる．その結果，顎関節の可動域の拡大，顎関節部と咀嚼筋の痛みの軽減・改善，咀嚼筋の耐性の向上等が期待できる．**Fig. 4-1** にリハビリトレーニングによる治療の流れを示す．

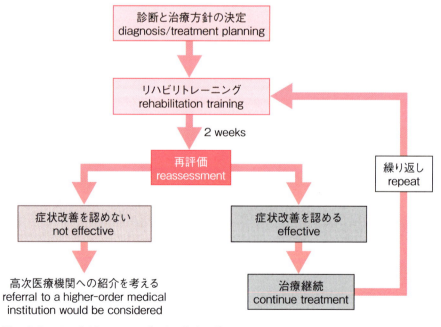

Fig. 4-1 リハビリトレーニングによる治療の流れ
Fig. 4-1 Treatment flow using rehabilitation training

1. Features and effects of rehabilitation training

The rehabilitation training is jaw opening exercise performed by patients themselves at home readily and non-invasively.

The purpose of this training is to increase joint mobility and reduce pain of TMJ and/or masticatory muscles. **Fig. 4-1** shows the flow of treatment using rehabilitation training.

2 リハビリトレーニングの種類と適応症
Types of rehabilitation training and their indications

リハビリトレーニングには，①関節可動化訓練，②筋伸展訓練，③開口維持訓練，④筋負荷訓練，⑤ガム咀嚼訓練がある．それぞれの適応症を踏まえて実施することが重要であるため，3章で紹介した医歯大式病型分類により治療方針を決定する(**Tab. 4-1**).

どの病型に対する治療でもリハビリトレーニングが主体になるが，クリック発現から2週間以内の症例(CE)では関節円板復位訓練を，ロックから2週間以内の症例(LE)にはマニピュレーション(関節円板整位術)を行う場合もある．変形性顎関節症に関しては，対応した特異的な治療方法はなく，関節可動化訓練などで十分な顎関節の可動域が得られれば，変形が改善することが多い．

1) 関節可動化訓練 (Fig. 4-2)

【対象となる病態】 A，AM，CE，CP，IL，LE，LC

顎関節の運動時痛の軽減と可動域の拡大を目的とする開口訓練であり，顎関節雑音(クリック)時の痛みの改善にも効果がある．

Tab. 4-1 各病型に対するリハビリトレーニングの選択
Tab. 4-1 Selection of rehabilitation training for each disease type

病型分類　type	リハビリトレーニング　rehabilitation training
M: 筋痛　myalgia	筋伸展訓練　muscle stretching exercise
MA/AM: 筋痛＋関節痛　myalgia+arthralgia	筋伸展訓練，関節可動化訓練　muscle stretching exercise, joint mobilization exercise
A: 関節痛　arthralgia	関節可動化訓練，開口維持訓練　joint mobilization exercise, open-mouth holding exercise
CE: クリック初期　early click	関節可動化訓練(状態に応じて関節円板復位訓練)　joint mobilization exercise (disc reduction exercise depending on conditions)
CO: クリック単独　click only	病態説明と経過観察　explanation of current condition and follow-up
CP: クリック＋痛み　click+pain	開口維持訓練，関節可動化訓練　open-mouth holding exercise, joint mobilization exercise
IL: 間欠ロック　intermittent lock	関節可動化訓練　joint mobilization exercise
LE: ロック初期　early lock	マニピュレーション，関節可動化訓練　manipulation, joint mobilization exercise
LC: 慢性ロック　chronic lock	関節可動化訓練　joint mobilization exercise

顎関節に問題を抱えている場合，痛みを全く伴わない開口訓練は効果がないが，リハビリテーション目的であってもいきなり強制的に大開口をさせると患者に不要な苦痛を与えることになるので，避けるべきである．十分な準備体操→適切な開口訓練→整理体操の流れでリハビリトレーニングを行うことが，最小限の副作用で最大限の効果を得るためのポイントである．

　訓練時および直後の痛みは避けられないが，患者にはその痛みをある程度我慢してもらわなければならない．患者が不安になることもあるかもしれないが，痛みを避けた訓練では症状の改善は全く期待できないことをよく説明する必要がある．痛みをこらえた訓練の先に症状の軽快が待っていることをよく理解してもらい，患者と二人三脚で治療を進めていく．そのためには適宜，鎮痛薬の使用による適切な痛みの管理と定期的な症状確認，必要に応じて訓練方法の再指導などの介入が必要となり，十分な説明を行って患者の理解を得，信頼関係を醸成することが重要である．

2) 筋伸展訓練 (Fig. 4-2)

【対象となる病態】M，MA

　咀嚼筋を伸展増大させることにより，咀嚼筋痛の改善を図る訓練である．顎関節痛を併発している場合は，顎関節の可動化訓練を兼ねることとなる．

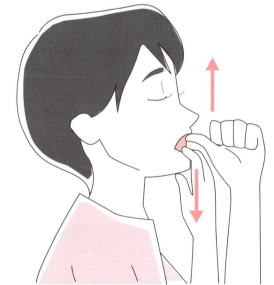

関節可動化訓練・筋伸展訓練（訓練動作は同じ）

① **準備体操**
　・痛みが生じない範囲で10回程度，軽く口を開け閉めする．
　・この時，口の中には何も入れないようにする．
　・開口量は下顎頭の前方滑走が生じない範囲，閉口は上下歯列の咬頭接触が起きない程度を目安とする．

② **訓練**
　・できるかぎり大きく開口する．開口障害や痛みを伴う場合は自力による大開口が困難なので，徒手によるアシストを行う．
　・顔を少し上に向け，利き手の示指，中指，薬指を下顎前歯の切縁にかけて下顎を前下方に押し下げるようにして強制開口を行う．
　・反対の手の拇指を上顎前歯に添えて両手で開大するように行うと，効果的に強制開口を行うことができる．
　・この時，できるだけ痛みを我慢して，痛みが生じた開口量からさらに開大させることが肝心である．
　・この状態で30～60秒キープする（症状や状況によって調節するが，最初は30秒程度から始める）．

③ **整理体操**
　　上記の①を行う．

上記①～③を4回繰り返す＝1セット
1日に4セット行う（起床時，昼食後，夕食後，入浴中，入浴後等）

＊入浴中，入浴後は体が温まり，こわ張りが少ないことから，訓練を楽に行いやすい

Fig. 4-2 関節可動化訓練・筋伸展訓練（木野 2017より）[1]

方法は関節可動化訓練と同じであるが，閉口筋の伸展を意識して行う．筋肉が気持ちよく伸展するいわゆる「伸び」のような感覚を咬筋と側頭筋に与えるように行うとよい．

3）開口維持訓練（Fig. 4-3）
【対象となる病態】 A，CP

血流の改善により開口時痛が消失することを目的とした訓練である．指を使わなくても大きく開口することができ，開口時関節痛があるだけの症例に対し行う．

4）筋負荷訓練（Fig. 4-4）
【対象となる病態】 筋の易疲労性

長く開口障害が続くと咀嚼筋の筋力が低下し，開口障害の改善後も開口状態の維持が困難であったり，顎が疲れやすかったりする．筋負荷訓練は特定の病態に対して行うものではなく，このような筋力の低下による易疲労性を改善するためのアイソメトリックトレーニングである．

5）ガム咀嚼訓練（Fig. 4-5）
【対象となる病態】 咀嚼時の関節痛

顎関節症の発症初期に開口障害とともに認められる運動時関節痛は，開口障害の改善に伴い消失することが多い．しかし，開口訓練による適応（リモデリング）の結果，さらに前方へと移動した関節円板の後部結合組織が下顎頭により圧迫されて咀嚼時に関節痛を生じることがある．このような場合に，ガム咀嚼訓練を行うことで症状の改善が期待できる．ガムを噛んで関節円板後部結合組織に負荷をかけ，痛みの原因である毛細血管を消滅させることを目的としたトレーニングである．

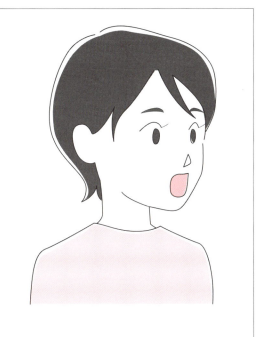

開口維持訓練

① **準備体操**
- 痛みが生じない範囲で10回程度，軽く口を開け閉めする．
- この時，口の中には何も入れないようにする．
- 開口量は下顎頭の前方滑走が生じない範囲，閉口は上下歯列の咬頭接触が起きない程度を目安とする．

② **訓練**
- 痛みをなるべく我慢しながら，できるかぎり大きく開口する．
- そのまま10秒キープする．慣れてきたら，時間を延ばす．

③ **整理体操**
上記の①を行う．

上記①～③を4回繰り返す＝1セット
1日に4セット行う（起床時，昼食後，夕食後，入浴中，入浴後等）

Fig. 4-3　開口維持訓練（木野 2017より）[1]

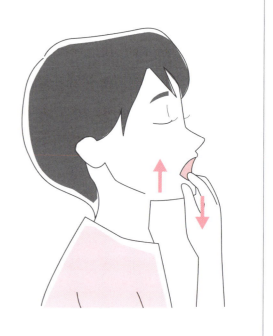

> **筋負荷訓練**
>
> ① **準備体操**
> ・痛みが生じない範囲で10回程度，軽く口を開け閉めする．
> ・この時，口の中には何も入れないようにする．
> ・開口量は下顎頭の前方滑走が生じない範囲，閉口は上下歯列の咬頭接触が起きない程度を目安とする．
>
> ② **訓練**
> ・顔を少し上に向けてから30 mm程度（二横指程度）開口し，利き手の示指，中指，薬指を下顎前歯の切縁にかけて下顎を前下方に押し下げる．
> ・指の力に拮抗するように自力で閉口動作を行い，開口量を維持したまま30〜60秒キープする（症状や状況によって調節するが，最初は30秒程度から始める）．
>
> ③ **整理体操**
> 上記の①を行う．
>
> 上記①〜③を4回繰り返す＝1セット
> 1日に4セット行う（起床時，昼食後，夕食後，入浴中，入浴後等）

Fig. 4-4 筋負荷訓練 (木野 2017より)[1]

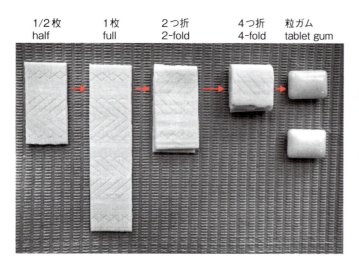

Fig. 4-5 ガム咀嚼訓練
咀嚼時に関節痛のある部位で，あえて痛みが出るようにガムを噛む．ガム1/2枚からスタートし，厚みや種類を順次変えていく．食事の時の痛みが消えれば訓練は終了

Fig. 4-5 Gum chewing training
Gum chewing is instructed to induce pain purposely at the sites of joint pain on mastication. The training starts with a half stick of gum and then continues with changing its folds or form gradually. This training is accomplished when no pain at meal has been achieved.

2. Types of rehabilitation training and their indications

Select treatment modality according to TMD classification by TMDU (**Tab. 4-1**).

1) Joint mobilization exercise (Fig. 4-2)

Goals: increase mouth-opening range, reduce pain.

Indications: A, AM, CE, CP, IL, LE, LC

Note: Feeling pain during/right after exercise is inevitable. Patients are expected to bear the pain because training that accompanies no pain is ineffective. Encourage the patient that

Chapter 4　顎関節症の病態治療

Joint mobilization exercise/ Muscle stretching exercise
(common actions are used for both exercises)

① **Warm-up**
・Open and close the mouth gently about ten times not to cause pain.
・Nothing should be kept in the mouth.
・The condylar protrusive movement should not occur when opening the mouth, nor occlusal contact when closing it.

② **Exercise**
・Open the mouth as wide as posibble. In case that trismus or pain hamper wide opening, assistance by fingers can be applied.
・Raise the head lightly, and put first, second and third fingers of the dominant hand on incisal edges of lower anterior teeth to push the mandible forward and downward. Add the thumb of the non-dominant hand on incisal edges of upper anterior teeth to force the mouth open effectively by both hands.
・Open the mouth wider against the onset of pain with the most possible patience.
・Hold the mouth open for 30–60 seconds. Start with 30 seconds which is adjusted depending on patients' conditions or situations.

③ **Cool-down**
　　Same as ①.

Repeat ①–③ 4 times：1 set.
Make 4 sets per day (on awakening, after lunch, after dinner, during or after bathing, etc.).

*Bathing warms the body and improves stiffness, which facilitates exercise.

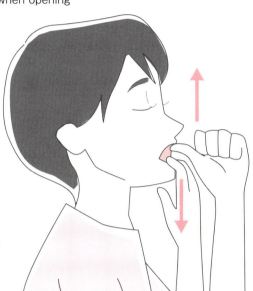

Fig. 4-2　Joint mobilization exercise/ Muscle stretching exercise

---

symptoms will improve after continuation of training with pain. Pain control with analgesics, periodical examination of symptoms and reinstruction (as needed) are required to build up a relationship of mutual trust.

2) **Muscle stretching exercise (Fig. 4-2)**
　　Goal: improve muscle pain.
　　Indications: M, MA

3) **Open-mouth holding exercise (Fig. 4-3)**
　　Goals: reduce jaw opening pain by increasing blood supply.
　　Indications: A, CP

4) **Muscle loading exercise (Fig. 4-4)**
　　Goal: increase muscle endurance to improve fatigability.
　　Indication: muscle fatigability.

5) **Gum chewing training (Fig. 4-5)**
　　Goal: degenerate microvessels which cause pain on mastication by loading force on TMJ.
　　Indication: joint pain on mastication.

Open-mouth holding exercise

① Warm-up
- Open and close the mouth gently about ten times not to cause pain.
- Nothing should be kept in the mouth.
- The condylar protrusive movement should not occur when opening the mouth, nor occlusal contact when closing it.

② Exercise
- Open the mouth as wide as possible bearing the most possible pain.
- Hold the mouth open for 10 seconds. Increase the length of time as getting used to it.

③ Cool-down
Same as ①.

Repeat ①-③ 4 times: 1 set.
Make 4 sets per day (on awakening, after lunch, after dinner, during or after bathing, etc.).

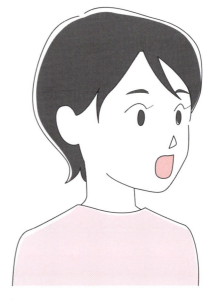

Fig. 4-3 Open-mouth holding exercise

Muscle loading exercise

① Warm-up
- Open and close the mouth gently about ten times not to cause pain.
- Nothing should be kept in the mouth.
- The condylar protrusive movement should not occur when opening the mouth, nor occlusal contact when closing it.

② Exercise
- Raise the head lightly, and open the mouth as wide as 30 mm (about 2 fingers' breadth), then put first, second and third fingers of the dominant hand on incisal edges of lower anterior teeth to push the mandible forward and downward.
- Make effort to close the mouth to countervail the force from fingers holding the mouth open for 30-60 seconds. Start with 30 seconds which is adjusted depending on patients' conditions or situations.

③ Cool-down
Same as ①.

Repeat ①-③ 4 times: 1 set.
Make 4 sets per day (on awakening, after lunch, after dinner, during or after bathing, etc.).

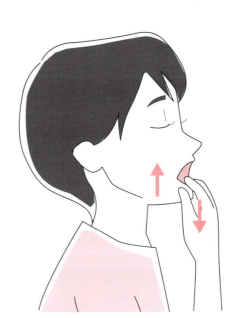

Fig. 4-4 Muscle loading exercise

Reference

1) 木野孔司 編著. 顎関節症のリハビリトレーニング. 医歯薬出版, 2017.

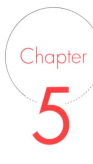

Chapter 5 顎関節症の病因診断

Etiological diagnosis of TMD

佐藤文明 *Fumiaki Sato*

顎関節症の病因の考え方 —単一病因説と多因子病因説—
Interpretations of pathogenesis of TMD –Single etiology and multifactorial etiology–

顎関節症は，以前は咬み合わせが唯一の原因であると考えられていた（単一病因説）．これは，顎関節症の原因は臼歯部の喪失であるとして，1930年代にアメリカの耳鼻科医Costenが歯科医に義歯を作らせ，症状が改善したと報告したことに始まる[1]．その後，咬合治療が盛んに行われるようになったが，症状改善は確実ではなく，さらに症状が悪化する患者もいた．

1970年代になると，咬み合わせだけでなく，いくつかの要因が重なって症状が出現するという多因子病因説が支持されるようになった[2]．顎関節や筋肉の弱さ，日常生活における癖や習慣，心理的ストレス等のさまざまな要因が積み重なり，その人がもつ耐久力を超えると顎関節症を発症するという考え方である．そして，これらの要因は寄与因子と呼ばれる．この多因子病因説は，**Fig. 5-1**のような寄与因子の積み木モデルを考えると理解しやすい．

多因子病因説の考え方に基づくと，同じ寄与因子をもっていても症状が出現する人とそうでない人がいることに対する説明がつく．また，咬合治療を受けて症状が改善した人と改善しない人がいることについても同様に理解しやすい．

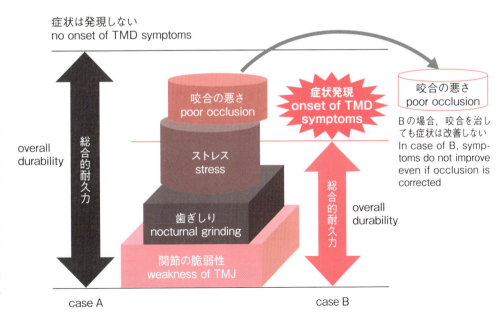

Fig. 5-1 積み木モデル
顎関節症の寄与因子を積み木に例えて説明すると，積み木がいくつも積み重なり患者の総合的な耐久力を超えてしまうことで，症状が発現する．治療ではいくつかの寄与因子をおろし，その患者のもつ総合的な耐久力の範囲内に収めることで改善を図る

Fig. 5-1 Building block model of multifactorial etiology

37

1. Interpretations of pathogenesis of TMD
   —Single etiology and multifactorial etiology—

Temporomandibular joint disorders (TMD) was once regarded to be caused by single factor, namely occlusion[1]. Currently, multifactorial etiology, that the accumulation of multiple factors causes TMD, is widely supported[2]. The onset depends on overall durability of each patient, which can be explained by a building block model (**Fig. 5-1**).

2 どの寄与因子を顎関節症治療のターゲットとするか？
Which contributing factors should be targeted for treatment of TMD?

2010年にAADR（American Academy of Dental Research：米国歯科研究学会）は顎関節症治療に対する基本声明[3]を発表し，顎関節症治療にあたっては，初期に咬合を触るような不可逆的治療ではなく保存療法を優先するべきであると述べている．

現在，顎関節症の寄与因子として**Fig. 5-2**に示すものが考えられているが，これらのなかで，AADRの基本声明に則り，われわれ一般歯科医が治療介入できるのはどれであろうか．解剖要因は生まれもったもので，改善するのは難しい．咬合要因については，咬合異常が顎関節症の原因であるとするエビデンスは弱く，顎関節症患者に観察される咬合異常は顎関節の病態に起因する二次的な結果であることも指摘されている．仮に咬合異常があっても，咬合治療は不可逆的であるため初期治療として行うことはできない．外傷要因は発症に関わっているが，予防的な対応は困難である．精神的要因については精神科医等とのリエゾン治療が必要であり，歯科医だけで対応するのは困難である（2章参照）．

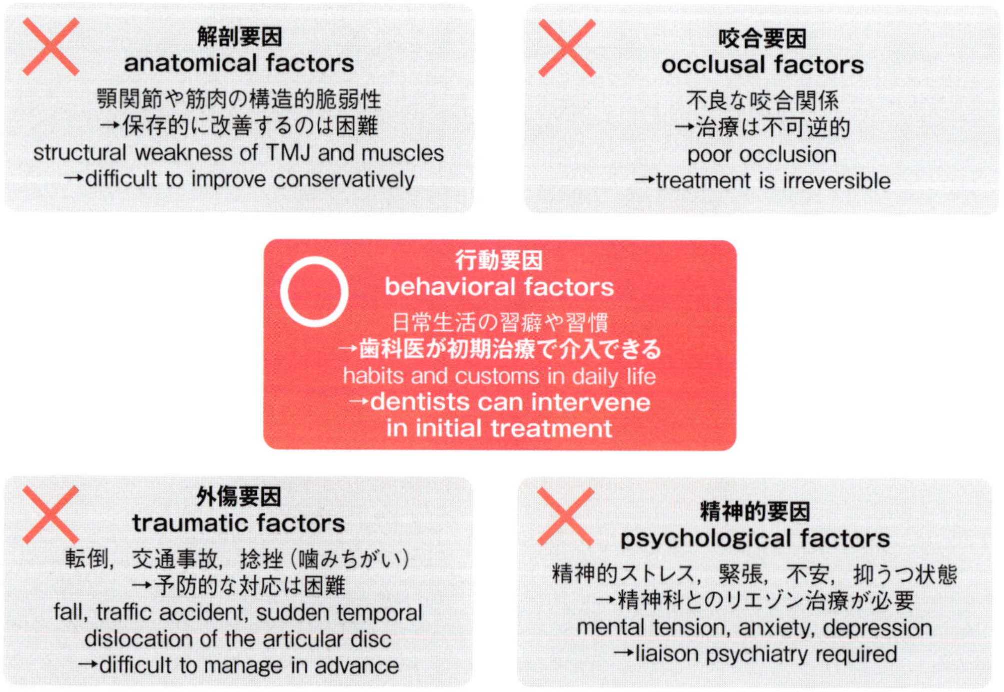

✗ 解剖要因 anatomical factors	✗ 咬合要因 occlusal factors
顎関節や筋肉の構造的脆弱性 →保存的に改善するのは困難 structural weakness of TMJ and muscles →difficult to improve conservatively	不良な咬合関係 →治療は不可逆的 poor occlusion →treatment is irreversible

○ 行動要因 behavioral factors
日常生活の習癖や習慣
→歯科医が初期治療で介入できる
habits and customs in daily life
→dentists can intervene in initial treatment

✗ 外傷要因 traumatic factors	✗ 精神的要因 psychological factors
転倒，交通事故，捻挫（噛みちがい） →予防的な対応は困難 fall, traffic accident, sudden temporal dislocation of the articular disc →difficult to manage in advance	精神的ストレス，緊張，不安，抑うつ状態 →精神科とのリエゾン治療が必要 mental tension, anxiety, depression →liaison psychiatry required

Fig. 5-2 顎関節症の発症，永続化に関する寄与因子と初期治療の可否
Fig. 5-2 Contributing factors which relate to the onset and the persistence of TMD

Tab. 5-1 顎関節症の発症に関与する行動要因

日常習癖	TCH（上下歯列接触癖），頬杖，不良姿勢，筆記具を咬む癖，爪咬み，携帯電話・スマートフォンの操作，うつぶせ読書，下顎突出癖，受話器を肩ではさむ姿勢，コンピュータゲーム
食事	硬固物咀嚼，ガム噛み，偏咀嚼
就寝時	ブラキシズム（クレンチング，グラインディング），睡眠不足，高い枕や固い枕の使用，手枕や腕枕，就寝時の姿勢
スポーツ	コンタクトスポーツ，球技，ウインタースポーツ，スキューバダイビング
音楽	楽器演奏，歌唱（カラオケ），発声練習
心理社会学的要因	緊張する仕事，多忙な生活，精密作業，重量物運搬，パソコン作業，対人関係の緊張

Tab. 5-1 Behavioral factors

habits, customs	TCH, resting chin on hand, poor posture, pencil biting, nail biting, long time operation of mobile phone, reading books while lying prone, jaw thrust, cradling the phone in neck, playing video game for a long time
meal	eating hard foods, gum chewing, mastication predominance
bedtime	bruxism (clenching, grinding), sleep deprivation, using a high and/or hard pillow, using arm/hand as pillow, sleep position
sports	contact sports, ball games, winter sports, scuba diving
music	playing instruments, singing or karaoke, vocal exercise
psychosocial factors	stressful work, busy life, detailed work, handling heavy materials, VDT operation, stress in personal relationships

Tab. 5-2 有痛性顎関節症患者における寄与因子の保有割合 (Sato 2006)[5]
Tab. 5-2 Prevalence (%) of contributing factors in TMD patients with pain

寄与因子　contributing factors	保有割合　prevalence (%)
偏咀嚼　mastication predominance	67.8
姿勢が悪い　poor posture	62.7
仕事が多忙　busy work	56.1
TCH（tooth contacting habit）	52.4
睡眠不足　sleep deprivation	47.6
長電話　long talk on the phone	47.6
家族による歯ぎしりの指摘　grinding pointed out by family	34.2

　したがって，比較的初期に介入しやすいのは行動要因ということになる．行動要因には，**Tab. 5-1** に示すようにさまざまな寄与因子が存在する．われわれが重視しているTCH（Tooth Contacting Habit：上下歯列接触癖）も，行動要因の一つとして考えている．

　しかし，これだけ多くの寄与因子のなかで，顎関節症患者の大多数がもっている寄与因子が何であるかは不明であったため，東京医科歯科大学顎関節治療部，顎顔面外科，東京慈恵会医科大学歯科の多施設共同で，2000年に大規模な調査を行った[4]．有痛性の顎関節症患者229名に対し，34項目にわたる因子について調査した結果，TCHは52.4％と半数以上の患者に認められた[5]（**Tab. 5-2**）．

その後，われわれの研究で，顎関節症の寄与因子としてTCHが症状に関連することが確認されたため[5]，われわれは顎関節症治療の主体にTCH是正訓練（病因に対する治療）を加え，リハビリトレーニング（病態に対する治療）と組み合わせて行うようになった（**Fig. 1-1**；9頁）．そして，TCHを是正することにより顎関節症の治療成果は飛躍的に向上した．

2. Which contributing factors should be targeted for treatment of TMD?

Factors currently assumed to contribute to TMD onset are shown in **Fig. 5-2**. In 2010, AADR (American Academy of Dental Research) suggested to prioritize conservative therapies over irreversible treatments, such as occlusal adjustment, at initial phase of TMD treatment[3]. Conservative therapies employed here target etiology and pathological condition in parallel. Upon approaching to etiology, behavioral factors shown in **Tab. 5-1** are manageable. Among these factors, those shown in **Tab. 5-2** are popular in TMD patients. Particularly, TCH (tooth contacting habit) is an extremely noticeable factor[4,5].

3 TCHとは
Tooth contacting habit

1) TCHの定義

TCHという用語は，前述した顎関節症の寄与因子を探る共同研究の際に，東京医科歯科大学顎関節治療部部長であった木野孔司先生と東京慈恵会医科大学歯科学教室教授であった杉崎正志先生により提唱された．

TCHの定義は「**安静時（非機能時）においても上下の歯が接触し続ける習癖**」である．本来，ヒトでは安静時に上下の歯は接触せず，1～3 mm程度の安静空隙が存在する．上下の歯は咀嚼，発話，嚥下などの機能時に瞬間的に接触するのみで，その接触時間は積算しても1日平均17.5分であると報告されている[6]．

一方，非機能時にも顎関節を含めた顎口腔系にはさまざまな力が加わっている．TCHも非機能的運動に含まれるが，日中のクレンチングとは別のカテゴリーとして考えている（**Fig. 5-3**）．

2) 日中のクレンチングとどう違うのか？

従来から夜間のクレンチング，グラインディングは顎関節症の原因の一つとして認識されてきた．しかし，日中のクレンチングについては，医療面接の際に「くいしばりや咬みしめはしていない」と答える患者が多く，調査が難しかった．「くいしばり」と聞いて患者がイメージするのはかなり強い力で咬む行為であり，日常生活ではそのようなことをしている意識はないものと考えられる．Nishiyamaらは，くいしばりと聞いて患者がイメージする力の大きさは，平均で最大咬合力の約70％であったと報告している[7]．

歯を強く咬みしめるクレンチングを行うと，筋の疲労感や鈍重感を引き起こし，その後も継続すると筋に痛みが生じる．しかし，このような強い咬みしめは筋血流量の減少と筋肉代謝の変化による痛みのため，長くても2～5分程度しか続けることはできないといわれている[8,9]．

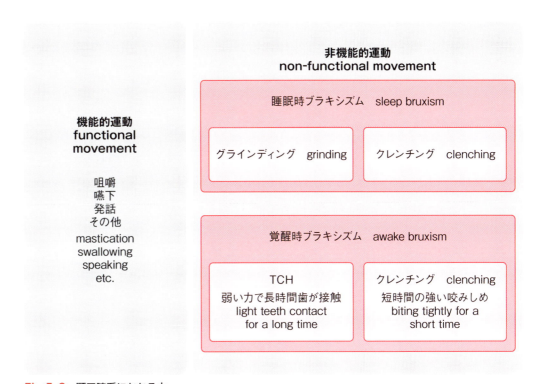

Fig. 5-3 顎口腔系にかかる力
Fig. 5-3 Force loaded on stomatognathic system

　一方，われわれが提唱しているTCHは歯を接触させ続けることであり，決して強く咬みしめることではない．
　Farellaらは，種々の力で疲労や痛みを感じるまで咬み続けられる時間を計測し，最大咬合力の40％の力では1.4分しか咬み続けられなかったのに対し，TCHを想定できる7.5％の咬合力では，157.2分もの長時間咬み続けることができたと報告している．さらに，40％の力では翌日に咬筋の圧痛は認めなかったが，7.5％の力では翌日も咬筋の圧痛が認められ，弱い力の持続が顎口腔系に影響を及ぼすことが示されている[10]．これらのことから，クレンチングと違い弱い力が継続してかかるTCHにはいっそうの注意が必要と考えられる．

3) TCHは気づきにくい

　医療面接で患者から話を聴くと，長時間TCHを続けている人が多い．歯の接触時間を調査した研究では，サンプリングした時間の45～72.9％で歯が接触していたことが報告されており[11]，弱い力であるため患者自身が習癖に気づいていないと考えられる．歯を接触させる習癖そのものを知らず，こちらからの問いかけで初めて気づき，「普段，歯は接触しているものだと思っていました」と言う人も少なくない．
　TCHのような弱い力が継続して作用していると，当初はその疲労感に気づかないが，長時間作用した負荷が積算した結果，疲労しきった状態で気づくことになる．気づきにくい分，TCHのほうがクレンチングよりも積算した顎口腔系への負荷は大きくなる可能性がある．このようなことから，患者には「クレンチングは長く続けることが難しく，痛みや疲労のため気づく可能性があるが，長時間続けられるTCHはなかなか気づけないのでより悪い」と説明している．

3. Tooth contacting habit

TCH is defined as "a habit of keeping upper and lower teeth in contact even at rest (non-functionally)". Naturally, in human beings, upper and lower teeth do not come into contact at rest, and interocclusal rest space of about 1-3 mm exists. Upper and lower teeth momentarily touch each other during functional movements, such as chewing, pronouncing, and swallowing. It is reported that total functional contact time is, on average, 17.5 minutes per day[6].

Clenching, which exhibits strong force, lasts for only 2-5 minutes[8,9]. On the other hand, TCH introduced here means persistent contact of teeth, rather than strong biting (**Fig. 5-3**).

A study demonstrated that 7.5% of maximum occlusal force equivalent to TCH continued as long as 157.2 minutes. As persistent weak force could affect stomatognathic system[10], extra attention should be paid to TCH which places a weak load continuously.

4 顎関節症の寄与因子としてのTCH
TCH as a contributing factor of TMD

1) TCHと顎関節症の症状との関わり

TCHが顎関節症の寄与因子であることを最初に明らかにしたのは，前述した2000年の多施設共同研究である．初診時に痛みが4カ月以上継続していた229名を選び，症状が発現してから来院するまでの間に痛みが軽くなっているグループと，痛みが不変もしくは悪化しているグループに分け，ロジスティック回帰分析を行ったところ，TCHがあると痛みが不変もしくは悪化する確率が約2倍になるという結果が出た．この解析から，TCHが症状の維持継続に関与する可能性が示された（**Fig. 5-4**）．

また他の寄与因子との関わりを調べてみると，TCHをもっている可能性は，偏咀嚼をする患者では2.8倍，精密作業に従事している患者では2.2倍と，高い関連性が示唆された[5]（**Fig. 5-5**）．

では，TCHはどのように顎関節症の症状と関連するのであろうか？閉口筋の筋電位を測定した研究によると，閉口時に上下の歯が接触している状態では，咬みしめを行っていなくても高い筋電位が記録され，閉口筋は活動している[12]．TCHが顎関節症の症状を引き起こすのは，このような閉口筋の活動が長時間続くことによるものであろうと推測される．最大咬合力の10％程度の力で持続的に咬み続ける影響を調べた研究でも，筋活動量が増加し，疲労感の増加がみられている[13]．

長時間のTCHの持続は，顎関節や閉口筋に絶えず過剰な負担をかけ，筋疲労や筋痛，さらには顎関節を絶えず圧迫することで関節内の血液循環を阻害し，結果として顎関節内の摩擦抵抗が増大して関節の痛みが引き起こされる可能性があると考えている（**Fig. 5-6**）．

2) TCHを保有する人の割合

有痛性顎関節症患者におけるTCHの保有割合は，前述した2000年の研究[5]では52.4％であり（**Fig. 5-7**），さらに2003年の調査[15]では77％を超えるなど，多数の人がこの習癖をもっていることが明らかになった．

従属変数：痛みの改善/不変・悪化
ロジスティック回帰分析結果
dependent variable: pain improved/ unchanged or deteriorated
results from logistic regression analysis

因子 contributing factors	オッズ比 odds ratio	95%信頼区間 95% CI	p値 p-value
年齢 age	1.030	1.006-1.055	0.014
TCH	1.944	1.020-3.704	0.043

TCHがあると，痛みが不変もしくは悪化する確率が約2倍になる
With TCH, probability that pain get unchanged or worsened becomes twice as high.

従属変数：TCHあり/なし
ロジスティック回帰分析結果
dependent variable: TCH（＋）/（－）
results from logistic regression analysis

因子 contributing factors	オッズ比 odds ratio	95%信頼区間 95% CI	p値 p-value
偏咀嚼 mastication predominance	2.802	1.400-5.606	0.004
精密作業に従事 detailed work	2.195	1.028-4.688	0.042

偏咀嚼をする人はTCHをもっている可能性が2.8倍，精密作業をしている人ではTCHをもっている可能性が2.2倍になる
With mastication predominance, the probability of having TCH is 2.8 times as high, and 2.2 times with detailed work.

Fig. 5-4　TCHと痛みの関わり
Fig. 5-4　Relation between TCH and pain

Fig. 5-5　TCHと他の寄与因子との関わり
Fig. 5-5　Relation between TCH and other contributing factors

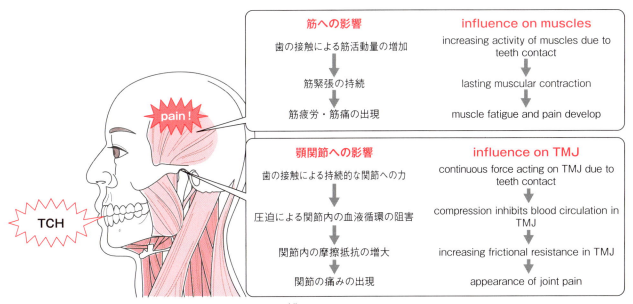

Fig. 5-6　TCHが筋や顎関節へ及ぼす影響 (佐藤 2011より)[14]
Fig. 5-6　Influence of TCH on muscles and TMJ

　　一方，企業の一般成人を対象とした調査では，TCHの保有割合は21％であった[16]．また，われわれが一般中学生955名の検診時に行った調査では，17.2％であった[17]（**Fig. 5-8**）．この調査では，顎関節症の症状のある生徒に限れば28.9％がTCHをもっており，TCHと顎関節症の症状との関連性が示唆される（**Fig. 5-9**）[17]．

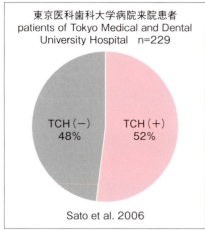

Fig. 5-7 顎関節症患者におけるTCH保有割合[5]
Fig. 5-7 Prevalence (%) of TCH in TMD patients with pain

Fig. 5-8 一般集団におけるTCH保有割合[16,17]
Fig. 5-8 TCH prevalence in general population

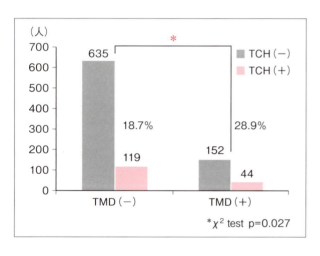

Fig. 5-9 TCHと顎関節症の症状との関わり
顎関節症の症状を有するグループでは，TCHのある割合が有意に高かった（佐藤 2014より）[17]
Fig. 5-9 Relation between TCH and TMD symptoms

4. TCH as a contributing factor of TMD

In 2000, we conducted a multicenter collaborative research. It revealed that the probability that the pain would get unchanged or worsened was approximately twice as high when TCH was accompanied. This result suggests the possibility that TCH contributes to the persistency of symptoms (**Fig. 5-4**). Considering the relation between TCH and other contributing factors, patients with mastication predominance and those who were engaged in detailed work[5] were likely to have TCH (**Fig. 5-5**).

It is supposed that long-lasting TCH overloads closure muscles continuously, resulting in muscle fatigue and muscle pain. Moreover, there is a possibility that persistent compression on TMJ interferes with local blood circulation, resulting in increasing frictional resistance in the temporomandibular joint, which leads to joint pain (**Fig. 5-6**).

In **Fig. 5-7** and **Fig. 5-8**, high prevalence of TCH is demonstrated[5,16,17]. In addition, positive association between TCH and temporomandibular joint symptoms is suggested in **Fig. 5-9**[17].

5 TCHはどのように定着するのか？
How does TCH become established?

1) TCHを行う状況

われわれの調査では精密作業時にTCHを行っている可能性が高いという結果が得られているが，医療面接で実際に患者から話を聴いても，やはりパソコン (PC) の長時間使用や，趣味等で集中して行う作業の際にTCHを行っている可能性が高い (**Fig.5-10**). PCの使用時間が2時間増加すると，顎関節症の症状をもつ可能性が2.23倍になるとの報告もある[18]. 予定の決められた集中作業で咬筋の活動が増えるとの研究もあり[19]，集中した作業中にTCHが継続しているためと考えられる．

また，以前よりストレスとクレンチングの関係が示唆されているが，現代社会では常に，会社や学校等，社会的な場所でさまざまなストレスにさらされている．ストレスを感じた時に咬みしめる動作をすることで，ストレスをコントロールするコーピングを行っているとも考えられる．もともと獲得行動としてTCHをもっている人が，緊張や忙しさによってTCHなどの習癖行動が増強されていると推測される[20,21].

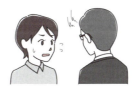
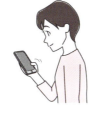
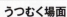
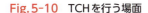

Fig.5-10　TCHを行う場面
Fig.5-10　Situations involving TCH

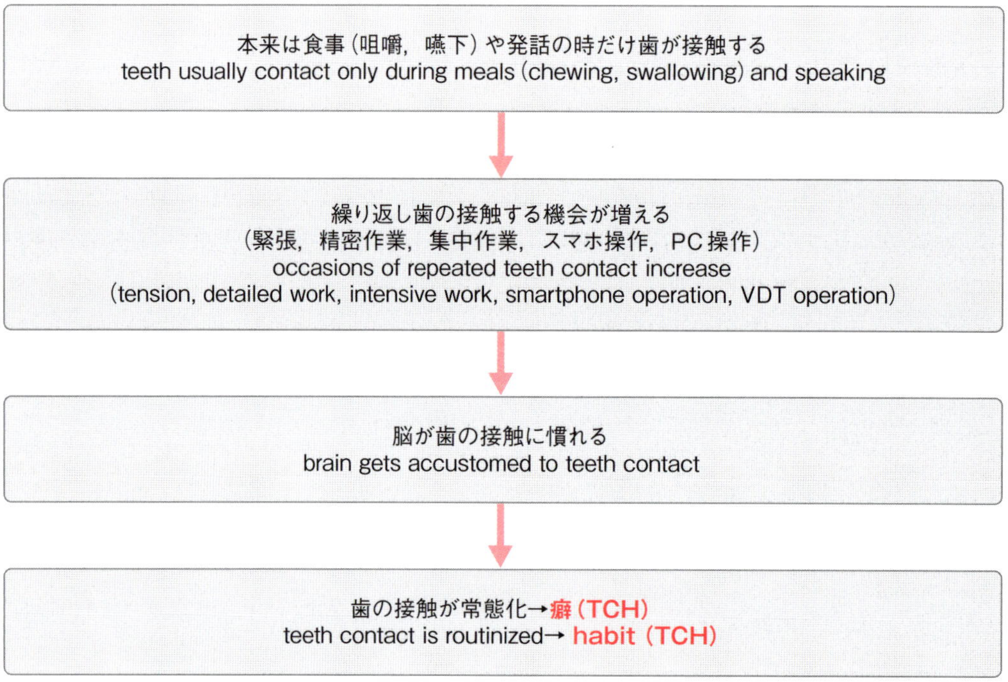

```
┌─────────────────────────────────────────────────────────┐
│ 本来は食事（咀嚼，嚥下）や発話の時だけ歯が接触する          │
│ teeth usually contact only during meals (chewing,        │
│ swallowing) and speaking                                 │
└─────────────────────────────────────────────────────────┘
                          ↓
┌─────────────────────────────────────────────────────────┐
│ 繰り返し歯の接触する機会が増える                          │
│ （緊張，精密作業，集中作業，スマホ操作，PC操作）           │
│ occasions of repeated teeth contact increase             │
│ (tension, detailed work, intensive work, smartphone      │
│ operation, VDT operation)                                │
└─────────────────────────────────────────────────────────┘
                          ↓
┌─────────────────────────────────────────────────────────┐
│ 脳が歯の接触に慣れる                                      │
│ brain gets accustomed to teeth contact                   │
└─────────────────────────────────────────────────────────┘
                          ↓
┌─────────────────────────────────────────────────────────┐
│ 歯の接触が常態化→癖（TCH）                               │
│ teeth contact is routinized→ habit（TCH）               │
└─────────────────────────────────────────────────────────┘
```

Fig. 5-11 TCHが定着するプロセス
Fig. 5-11 Process of TCH establishment

2）なぜTCHをもつようになるのか？

　TCHをもっている人は，どのようにしてその癖を獲得するのだろうか．もともとは食事等の機能時のみ歯が接触していたのが，**Fig. 5-10**のように緊張や集中する場面，うつむく姿勢等で歯を接触させる機会が増え，そのような状態が繰り返し継続していくことにより，歯を接触させることに脳が慣れてしまい，触れていることが普通の状態になってしまうのではないだろうか（**Fig. 5-11**）．

　本来，1日20分程度しか接触しないはずであるのに，何時間も接触させていることが常態化していれば，筋や関節も徐々に疲労し，さらにその状態が続けば痛みとして自覚するようになると考えられる．

5. How does TCH become established?

Our survey indicates that TCH is more likely to occur during detailed work, typically found in long period of VDT operation or devotion to hobbies (**Fig. 5-10**).

Normally, teeth contact occurs with functional activities such as chewing or speaking. However, as opportunities of teeth contact increases with tension, concentration, or slouching posture (**Fig. 5-10**)[20,21], repeating such situation gets the brain accustomed to the continuous teeth contact, and finally, makes it become habitual behavior (**Fig. 5-11**). Normal contact time should be less than 20 minutes a day. Therefore, if long-lasting habitual contact exists, muscles and joints become fatigued gradually. The prolonged fatigue has potential to develop pain.

6 TCHの診察と診断
Examination and diagnosis of TCH

　ここまで述べてきたように，TCHは多くの顎関節症患者の症状に関わりをもつことから，TCHを適確に診断し対応することができれば，治療効果は高いと思われる．しかし残念ながら，現在のところ客観的にTCHを判定する方法はない．ただし，臨床である程度推測することは可能であり，現在はいくつかの方法を組み合わせてTCHの判定を行っている．

1）問診によるTCHの判定
① 問診
　TCHの有無を調べたい場合には，巻末の付録No.3のような問診票に記入させることも一つの方法である．また，TCHが顎関節症の増悪要因として大きい場合には，日中，長時間にわたりTCHで力がかかり続けた結果，夕方に症状が出るケースが多い．起床時は症状がなく，夕方になると痛い，疲れる等の訴えがある場合はTCHの存在を疑う．これは夜間ブラキシズムのある人が起床時に咬みしめ感や痛み，疲労などを訴えるのとは対照的である．

② 閉眼判定法
　また，問診の際に，歯の接触について**Fig. 5-12**のような方法で患者に尋ねる．この方法の注意点として，TCHはない，もしくは弱いと判定した場合も，TCHを是正するトレーニング（詳細は6章参照）を行ってみると，患者が「やはりTCHがありました」と気づくことがあるため，その場だけで判断しないことが重要である．

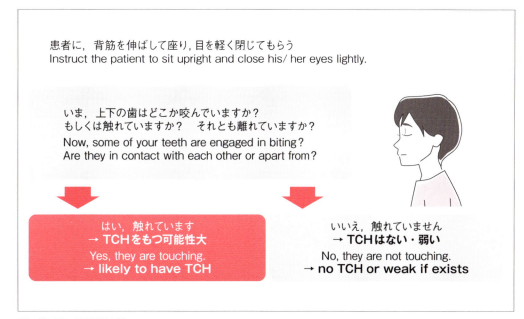

Fig. 5-12　閉眼判定法
Fig. 5-12　Eye closure method

2) 視診による判定法

① 咬筋部の観察

顔貌を観察し，咬筋の肥大がないか観察する．また問診中に患者が時折，咬みしめるような仕草をみせたり，頻繁に歯を合わせるような動作を行ったりして咬筋部を緊張させていないかもチェックする (**Fig. 5-13**).

② 舌圧痕，頰粘膜圧痕

口腔内所見として舌圧痕，頰粘膜圧痕がないかを観察する (**Fig. 5-13**)．気をつけなければいけないのは，舌圧痕や頰粘膜圧痕があるからといって，必ずしもTCHがあるという証拠とはならないことである．しかし，これらの所見は何らかの原因で下顔面領域の緊張状態が長いことをうかがわせるものであることから，他の方法との組み合わせで判定する．

3) 行動診察法

TCHの強い患者では，しばしば「唇を閉じてください」と言うと，一緒に上下の歯も接触させてしまう．これは幼少期から形成されている癖と思われるが，口唇を閉じた時に歯を離すことを同時に行う行動パターンができていないためである．このような患者では，口唇を閉じた状態で歯を離すように指示しても，違和感を覚えて持続が困難である．このような行動特性を利用した2つのテストを両方実施して，TCHの有無を判定する．

① LCTA (Lips Closed Teeth Apart：歯列離開) テスト (**Fig. 5-14**)

TCHのある患者では上下歯列が接触している状態のほうが楽であり，違和感が少ない．ファーストテストで判定できない場合，セカンドテストに移る．また，患者の動作をよく観察することも必要で，歯列を離すよう指示した際に口唇まで離れてしまうような場合はTCHがあると判定できる．

② LCTC (Lips Closed Teeth Contact：歯列接触) テスト (**Fig. 5-15**)

TCHのある患者では，弱い咀嚼筋の緊張が持続している．

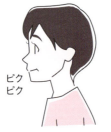
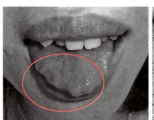
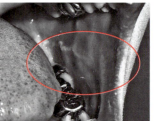

Fig. 5-13　視診によるTCHの判定法
Fig. 5-13　Inspection of TCH

Chapter 5 顎関節症の病因診断

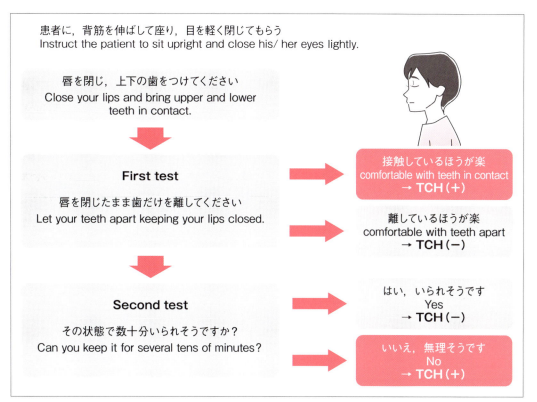

Fig. 5-14 歯列離開テスト (LCTA test)

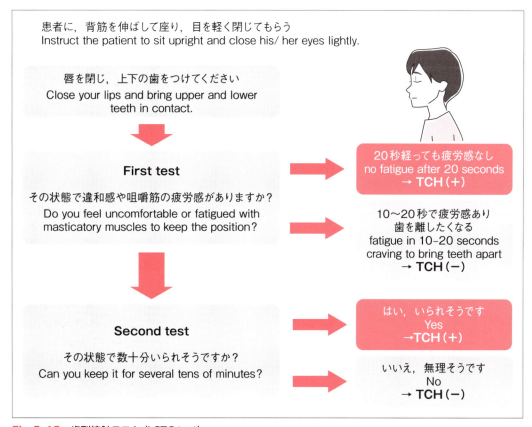

Fig. 5-15 歯列接触テスト (LCTC test)

この状態に慣れてしまっているために，筋を緊張させるように歯を接触させてもあまり違和感を覚えることなく継続できてしまう．この特性を利用し，TCHの有無を判定する．

6. Examination and diagnosis of TCH

1) TCH assessment by interview

① Medical interview

A medical questionnaire to check TCH is a useful instrument (Appendix No. 3). When patients have TCH as an etiological factor of TMD, their symptoms, such as pain or fatigue at joints and/or muscles, often appear in the evening, as a result of long-lasting force of TCH during all day long. Therefore, patients who complain of these symptoms in the evening rather than in the morning (after waking up) are suspected of having TCH.

② Eye closure method

In medical interview, ask the patient about teeth contact according to the procedure shown in **Fig. 5-12**. Even if TCH is assessed as negative or weak, some patients perceive TCH after correction training (see Chapter 6 for details). Definitive assessment should not be made at the first consultation.

2) Assessment by inspection

① Observation of the masseter (**Fig. 5-13**)

② Tongue indentation and buccal mucosa ridging (**Fig. 5-13**)

Keep in mind that these findings does not always testify TCH. However, they indicate existence of causes for persistent tension in the lower face.

3) Behavioral examination

Patients with significant TCH tend to bring their upper and lower teeth together when requested to close lips. In addition, they feel difficulty to keep teeth apart with lips closed. The following 2 tests adopting such behavioral features are useful to assess TCH.

① LCTA (Lips Closed Teeth Apart) test (**Fig. 5-14**)

Patients accompanying TCH feel comfortable and easy with the upper and lower teeth in contact with each other. In case of the first test turned out ineffective, move on to the second test. Also, it is necessary to carefully observe the behavior of the patient. Those whose lips open along with teeth separation are assessed to have TCH.

② LCTC (Lips Closed Teeth Contact) test (**Fig. 5-15**)

In patients with TCH, weak tension of masticatory muscles is sustained. They can continue keeping their teeth in contact with each other easily because they are accustomed to this condition. This characteristic is utilized to assess the presence or absence of TCH.

References

1) Costen JB. A syndrome of ear and sinus symptoms dependent upon disturbed function of the temporomandibular joint. *Ann Otol Rhinol Laryngol*. 1934; **43**: 1-15.

2) Weinberg LA. Temporomandibular dysfunctional profile: a patient-oriented approach. *J Prosthet Dent*. 1974; **32**: 312-325.

3) American Academy of Dental Research. AADR TMD policy statement revision approved by AADR Council 3/3/2010.

4) Kino K, Sugisaki M, Haketa T, et al. The comparison between pains, difficulties in function and associating factors of patients in subtypes of temporomandibular disorders. *J Oral Rehabil*. 2005; **32**: 315-325.

5) Sato F, Kino K, Sugisaki M, et al. Teeth contacting habit as a contributing factor to chronic pain in

patients with temporomandibular disorders. *J Med Dent Sci*. 2006; **53**: 103-109.
6） Graf H. Bruxism. *Dent Clin North Am*. 1969; **13**: 659-665.
7） Nishiyama A, Otomo N, Tsukagoshi K, Tobe S, Kino K. Magnitude of bite force that is interpreted as clenching in patients with temporomandibular disorders: A pilot study. *Dentistry*. 2014; S2: S2-004.
8） Lyons MF, Rouse ME, Baxandale RH. Fatigue and EMG changes in the masseter and temporalis muscles during sustained contractions. *J Oral Rehabil*. 1993; **20**(3): 321-331.
9） Christensen LV. Jaw muscle fatigue and pains induced by experimental tooth clenching: a review. *J Oral Rehabil*. 1981; **8**(1): 27-36.
10） Farella M, Soneda K, Vilmann A, et al. Jaw muscle sorenesss after tooth-clenching depends on force level. *J Dent Res*. 2010; **89**(7): 717-721.
11） Glaros AG, Williams K, Lausten L, et al. Tooth contact in patients with temporomandibular disorders. *Cranio*. 2005; **23**(3): 188-193.
12） Rugh JD, Drago CJ. Vertical dimension: A study of clinical rest position and jaw muscle activity. *J Prosthet Dent*. 1981; **45**: 670-675.
13） Svensson P, Burgaard A, Schlosser S. Fatigue and pain in human jaw muscles during a sustained, low-intensity clenching task. *Arch Oral Biol*. 2001; **46**(8): 773-777.
14） 佐藤文明．寄与因子としてのTCHの重要性と他の因子との関連性．歯界展望．2011；**117**（3）：416-419.
15） 木野孔司，杉崎正志，羽毛田 匡ほか．顎関節症に対する保存治療の変化による症状改善効果．日顎誌．2007；**19**（3）：210-217.
16） 西山　暁，木野孔司，杉崎正志ほか．企業就労者の顎関節症症状に影響を及ぼす寄与因子の検討．日顎誌．2010；**22**（1）：1-8.
17） 佐藤文明．学校歯科健康診断における顎関節調査法の検討とその疫学的特徴．東京都学校歯科医会会誌．2014；**77**：15-21.
18） Nishiyama A, Kino K, Sugisaki M, et al. A survey of influence of work environment on temporomandibular disorders-related symptoms in Japan. *Head Face Med*. 2012; **8**: 24.
19） Nicholson RA, Townsend DR, Gramling SE. Influence of a scheduled-waiting task on EMG reactivity and oral habits among facial pain patients and no-pain controls. *Appl Psychophysiol Biofeedback*. 2000; **25**(4): 203-219.
20） 杉崎正志，高野直久，木野孔司ほか．東京都内就労者における質問票による顎関節症有病率調査．日顎誌．2008；**20**（2）：127-133.
21） Nishiyama A, Kino K, Sugisaki M, et al. Influence of phychosocial factors and habitual behavior in temporomandibular disorder-related symptoms in a working population in Japan. *Open Dent J*. 2012; **6**: 240-247.

Chapter 6 顎関節症の病因治療

Etiological treatment of TMD

佐藤文明 *Fumiaki Sato*

1 顎関節症の病因治療の概念
Concept of etiological treatment of TMD

1）治療対象とする寄与因子の決定

　5章では，顎関節症の病因論として，いくつかの寄与因子が重なって症状が出現する多因子病因説を積み木モデルで説明した．病因治療の要は，積み木のように重なった寄与因子が何であるかを特定し，それを取り除くことによって患者のもつ関節や筋肉の耐久力の中に収めることである（**Fig.6-1**）．

　しかし，これらの寄与因子は通常，それ一つで顎関節症の症状を引き起こすほどの大きい影響強度があるわけではなく，また患者によって寄与因子の種類や大きさはさまざまである．寄与因子の顎関節症への影響強度を測定することも難しいため，取り除けそうな寄与因子をピックアップしてアプローチする以外に方法はない．

　5章で示した多くの寄与因子のうち，一般歯科医が積極的に介入できるのは行動要因である．行動要因をピックアップするには，巻末の付録No.3のような生活・行動要因調査票を用いるのもよい．寄与因子が抽出できたら，その中のどの因子を取り除くかを決めていく．その際，以下の点を考える必要がある（**Fig.6-1**）．

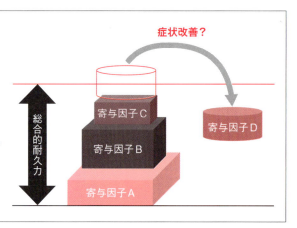

Fig.6-1 顎関節症の病因治療（積み木おろし治療法）
多因子疾患である顎関節症の治療では，いくつかの寄与因子（積み木）をおろし，患者のもつ総合的耐久力の範囲内に収めるような治療戦略が必要

① 顎関節症の症状が悪化する時に関係している寄与因子か？
② その寄与因子を取り除くことで，何か害を及ぼさないか？
③ 患者の生活の中で取り除くことが可能な因子か？

これらに合致する寄与因子として，われわれはTCH（Tooth Contacting Habit：上下歯列接触癖）を重要視しており，最初に取り除く因子であると考えている．

2）なぜTCHを最初に取り除くのか？

TCHを最初に取り除くべきであると考えるのは，TCHが顎関節症患者の半数以上に認められる寄与因子であることに加え，TCH是正はそれを行うことによって他の問題を引き起こさない可逆的な治療だからである．どの寄与因子がどの程度影響しているのかがわからない多因子疾患の顎関節症治療では，TCH是正による力のコントロールを行いながら，その反応をみつつ，他の原因も探っていく方向性が大切であると考えられる．

1. Concept of etiological treatment of TMD

1) Determination of contributing factors to be treated

The essence of etiological treatment of temporomandibular disorder (TMD) is to identify contributing factors and turn them down in the durability of the joint and muscle of each patient by removing some of them (**Fig.6-1**).

Among many contributing factors shown in Chapter 5, it is the behavioral factors in which general dentists can proactively intervene. Once the contributing factors are extracted using such questionnaires shown in Appendix No. 3, decide factor(s) to remove.

2) Why should TCH be removed first?

TCH is a contributing factor found in more than half of TMD patients, and correction of TCH is a reversible procedure which never cause other problems. In multifactorial diseases, it is unknown to what extent a certain contributing factor influences. Therefore, it is important to begin with approaching TCH as a possible etiology and look for other probable causes while observing changes in the patient's condition induced by TCH correction training.

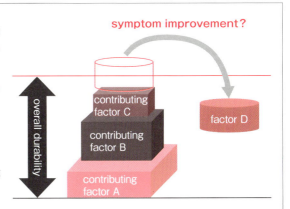

Fig.6-1 Etiological treatment of TMD: lowering building blocks

2 TCH是正訓練にあたっての注意点
Important points of TCH correction training

　TCHを是正するにあたっては，以下のことに注意する（Fig. 6-2）．

① TCHは無意識に行っているため，本人は気づけない

　癖として無意識に行っていることは，自分自身ではなかなか気づかず，他人に指摘されて初めて気づくことも多い．さらに，歯を接触させ続けることが顎口腔系に悪い影響を及ぼすことを知らなければ，TCHに気づくきっかけもないだろう．歯が接触していることが当たり前という状況を変える必要がある．ただし，この習癖について患者に教育しても，適切な方法を用いなければやめさせることは難しい．

② TCHは歯を接触させ続けることが問題を引き起こす

　TCHが咬みしめやくいしばりと異なることは，5章で述べたとおりである．弱い力であっても歯を接触させ続けることが問題であり，接触時間が長いほど筋や関節の負荷は増大する．

　咀嚼，嚥下，発話などの正常な機能時以外にも，緊張している時，重い物を持つ時，運動している時などに歯の接触は起こる．しかし，短時間で単発の歯の接触（teeth contact）であり，その人の耐久力の範囲内であれば，問題とはならないであろう．それが繰り返し行われ（repetition of teeth contact），さらに常態化すると習癖（TCH）となる．そうなると，時間経過とともにTCHの作用が累積し，何らかの臨床症状が出現する場合がある（Fig. 6-3）．

　どの程度の接触時間で症状が現れるかは，個体の耐久力によるため，寄与因子であるTCHがあったとしても，顎関節症の症状がない場合は問題とならない．

③「TCHは悪いのでやめなさい」と注意しても，患者はやめられない

　TCH是正の際に一番してはいけないことは，「TCHは顎関節症に悪いのでやめなさい」，「歯を離すようにしてください」などと言葉で注意することである．これでやめられる人はまずいない．

1	無意識で行っている癖であるため，本人が気づいていない． TCHを知らないため，歯の接触が悪いという認識がない． Because the habit is practiced unconsciously, patients are not aware of TCH. Ignorance of TCH hinders them from realizing that teeth contact is harmful.
2	上下の歯が長時間接触していることが問題を引き起こす． Long-lasting contact of upper and lower teeth causes problems.
3	「歯を離してください」という指導だけでは改善できない． 行動を伴った習慣逆転法を用いる． Verbal instruction to set teeth apart is not effective. Use habit reversal method to modify patient's behavior.

Fig. 6-2　是正訓練にあたって注意すべきTCHの特徴
Fig. 6-2　Features of TCH which requires correction training

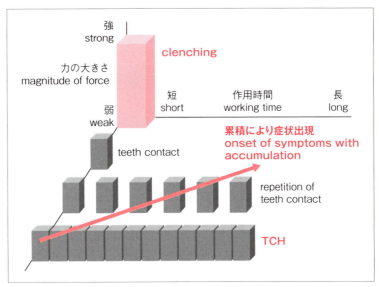

Fig. 6-3 TCHとクレンチングの相違点
歯の接触が常態化して，時間経過とともにTCHの作用が累積すると，臨床症状が出現する

Fig. 6-3 Difference between TCH and clenching

この癖を修正するには，習慣逆転法という心理療法の一手法を使うことが有効である．習慣逆転法により，患者自身が常態化しているTCHに気づき，より問題の少ない単発のteeth contactへと行動を変容させることを目標とする．

2. Important points of TCH correction training

In correcting TCH, following attention should be paid (**Fig. 6-2**).
① Unconscious TCH is hardly perceived

It is critical to inform the patient that TCH adversely affects the stomatognathic system, and such a bad habit should be rectified. However, even if patients are educated about this habit, it is difficult for them to stop it unless appropriate methods are provided.

② Long-lasting teeth contact induces problems

Even with weak force, keeping teeth in contact increases the burden on the muscles and joints, since the contact time prolongs. When repetition of teeth contact turns into a habit, baneful influences of TCH accumulates over time, and some clinical symptoms may occur (**Fig. 6-3**).

③ Verbal instruction to stop TCH is rarely effective

To correct this habit, a method of psychotherapy called habit reversal should be employed. The fundamental of this method is that notifying the existence of TCH helps to achieve behavior modification.

3 習慣逆転法によるTCHの是正
Correction training of TCH by habit reversal method

1) 習慣逆転法とは

　習慣逆転法（habit reversal method）は行動変容法と呼ばれる心理療法の一手法であり，望ましくない習癖行動をもつ人に対して，その習癖行動の頻度を減らすために用いられる[1]．習癖自体は頻度や強度が極端にならないかぎり問題ではなく，治療の対象とはならない．しかし，習癖行動が高頻度で起こっている場合や強い強度で生じている場合には異常習癖として取り扱われ，治療的介入が必要となる．

　習慣逆転法は運動チック，吃音等の神経性習癖の治療に用いられている．神経性習癖とは，物や自分の身体の一部を繰り返し操作する行動をいい，髪の毛を抜く，指の皮を剝く等，手を使った行動が多いが，爪や唇を咬む，（日中に）歯ぎしりをする等，口に関連した行動も多い．

　習慣逆転法の実践には，**Fig.6-4**に示す3つのステップが必要である．まず，最初のステップは動機づけ（motivation strategy）と呼ばれ，習癖がどのようなもので，どのような状況で生じるか，そしてその習癖があることでいかに不自由や困難が生じるかを患者に理解させることから始まる．

　第2のステップは意識化訓練（awareness training）といい，習癖が生じている，あるいは生じる予兆があった時に，それを確認することを学習させる．これには，習癖を感知できるような訓練が必要である．

　第3のステップは競合反応訓練（competing response training）といい，習癖が生じるたびに，またその予兆があった時に先行して，競合反応を使用することを練習する．競合反応は，

---

1. 動機づけ　motivation strategy

習癖がどのような状況で生じるか，習癖がいかに不自由と困難を引き起こすか，理解させる．
Patients should understand the circumstances under which the habit occurs, and know the inconvenience and difficulty derived from TCH.

2. 意識化訓練　awareness training

習癖が出現していることに気づき，確認する．習癖を感知できるような訓練が必要．
Awareness and identification of ongoing TCH is required.
Training is necessary for the patient to perceive the habit.

3. 競合反応訓練　competing response training

習癖が生じるたびに，またその予兆があった時に先行して，競合反応を使用することを練習する．
競合反応は習癖行動と両立しない行動にする．
Practice to apply competing response in preparation for emergence of the habit or its sign.
Competing response refers to a behavior that is incompatible with the habitual behavior.

Fig.6-4　習慣逆転法
Fig.6-4　Habit reversal method

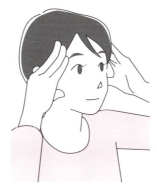

Fig.6-5 TCH是正訓練　ステップ1
Fig.6-5 TCH correction training: Step 1

習癖行動と両立しない行動とする．通常，患者が1～3分程度で行える，あまり目立たない行動をさせることが多い．

2) TCH是正訓練の実際

TCHは神経性習癖とみなすことができるため，習慣逆転法を用いた是正訓練が効果的である．次の3ステップで是正を試みる．

【ステップ1　動機づけ】(Fig.6-5)

まず，TCHという歯を接触させる行動が長時間続くことが，顎の関節や筋肉に悪い影響を与えていることを認識させる．歯を接触させている時間は，通常，1日の中で17.5分しかないことも患者に情報として伝える．それを聞いて，接触時間の短さに驚く患者も多い．

さらに親指と人差し指で咬筋と側頭筋を触らせ，口を開け閉めさせる．歯を接触させると筋が一緒に収縮する感覚を体験させることで，咬みしめていなくても筋肉を使っていることを実感させる．

【ステップ2　意識化訓練】(Fig.6-6)

TCHの行動を意識できるようにするには，無意識にやっているTCHを気づかせる方法をとる．「歯を離す」「リラックス」「力を抜く」などと書いた同じ色の貼り紙（リマインダー）を用意し，5分以上いる場所に10カ所以上貼る．視線を移せば，どこでも貼り紙があるという環境を作り出し，貼り紙を見た時にハッと気づくことが大切である．TCHをする可能性のある状況を情報として患者に知らせておくと，患者が効果的な場所を見つけやすい．パソコンの周囲，デスク周り，書類ホルダーなど目に留まりやすい場所に貼る．

渡邊らは，顎関節症患者における日中クレンチングの自覚度調査において，アンケートを重ねるうちに日中クレンチングに気づく機会が27％から39％，57％，67％と漸増することを報

Step 2　意識化訓練　awareness training

1. 同じ色の貼り紙（リマインダー）を用意し，自分が気づきやすい場所に貼る．
2. 貼り紙を見たら，上下の歯が接触しているかどうかを確認する．

- 貼り紙は最低でも10枚以上，目につきやすい場所や5分以上いる場所に貼る．
- 貼り紙を見た時に，ハッと気づくことが大切．

1. Post stickers (reminders) of same color on noticeable places.
2. When a sticker come into sight, check whether the upper and lower teeth are in contact.

- Ten reminders and more are to be posted on noticeable spots, or in places where patients stay for five minutes or more.
- Reminders should improve the level of awareness.

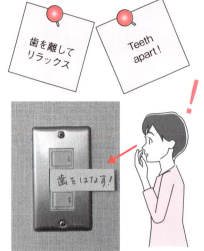

Fig. 6-6　TCH是正訓練　ステップ2
Fig. 6-6　TCH correction training: Step 2

Step 3　競合反応訓練　competing response training

1. 貼り紙を見た時に上下の歯が接触していたら，肩を大きく上げて，鼻から空気を吸い込む．
2. 一気に口から息を吐きながら，肩を落とし，全身の力を抜く．

- これらの動作を1回だけ行う．

1. If the upper and lower teeth are in contact when a reminder comes into sight, raise shoulders thoroughly and breathe in through the nose.
2. While breathing out through the mouth all at once, drop shoulders and relax the whole body, simultaneously.

- This sequence of actions should be done only once.

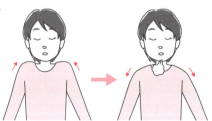

Fig. 6-7　TCH是正訓練　ステップ3
Fig. 6-7　TCH correction training: Step 3

告しており，繰り返し教育していくことにより習癖に気づく機会が増えることを裏づけている．さらに日中クレンチングに気づく場面は，当初はパソコン作業，仕事，読書であったりするが，調査を重ねるごとに考えごと，料理，食後の後片付けなどでも気づくようになると報告しており，繰り返しの患者教育が意識化につながるとしている[2]．

最初の貼り紙から1～2週間が経過すると，貼り紙が周りの景色と同化し，気づく効果がなくなるため，貼り紙の色を変えるとよい．

Chapter 6　顎関節症の病因治療

【ステップ3　競合反応訓練】(Fig.6-7)

　貼り紙を見たら，必ず上下の歯が接触しているか自己チェックをしてもらう．接触していた場合は，一度肩を大きく上げて，鼻から大きく息を吸い込み，その後，口から息を吐きながら肩を落とし，一気に脱力する．この時，できるだけ全身を脱力させることが重要である．この動作は，一度だけ行うよう指導する．

3. TCH correction training by habit reversal method

Habit reversal is a behavior modification method used in psychotherapy to reduce the frequency of undesirable habitual behavior[1].

It consists of three steps demonstrated in **Fig.6-4**.

【Step 1: Motivation strategy】(**Fig.6-5**)

At the beginning, get the patient to recognize that long-lasting teeth contact adversely affects jaw muscles and TMJ. Instruct the patient to open and close the mouth with her/his thumbs placed on the masseter and index fingers placed on the temporalis. The patient can feel the muscles contracted when teeth are brought into contact, which informs the patient that muscles are used even when strong-force-required activities like clenching are not practiced.

【Step 2: Awareness training】(**Fig.6-6**)

Bring the ongoing TCH up in consciousness. Prepare stickers of same color as reminders with messages, such as "teeth apart" "relax" "relieve tension of the shoulders", etc. Post them on ten and more spots—for example, around PC or on stationary products— at the place where patients stay for more than five minutes. Patients can easily conceive of effective spots for reminders if they are informed of the very likely situations that accompany TCH. Reminders should come into sight whenever the patient slides a glance to remind her/him of TCH. After 1-2 weeks, reminders become less effective as they assimilate surrounding things. This can be managed by changing the color of stickers.

【Step 3: Competing response training】(**Fig.6-7**)

When a reminder come into sight, the patient should check whether upper and lower teeth are in contact by her/himself. If teeth are in contact, raise shoulders thoroughly, breathe in deeply through the nose then breathe out through the mouth while dropping shoulders, and relax the whole body all at once. This sequence of actions should be done only once.

4　TCH是正の評価

Evaluation of TCH correction

1) TCH是正訓練の効果

　習慣逆転法でTCH是正訓練を行うと，初めのうちは貼り紙を見た後に「脱力しなければ」という意志が働き，脱力していたのが，次第に貼り紙を見たらすぐに脱力行動をとる条件反射が形成されていく．さらに，歯が接触している時の筋肉の軽い疲労感を自覚できるようになる(**Fig.6-8**)．そして，歯の接触から疲労感を自覚するまでの時間が徐々に短縮していき，歯が接触するとすぐに脱力する行動がとれるようになれば，TCHからは離脱できたと考えられる．

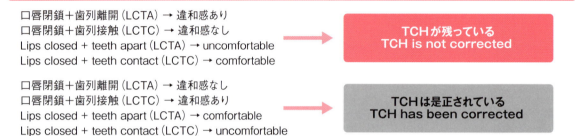

Fig. 6-8　TCH是正訓練の効果とその評価法
Fig. 6-8　Effect and evaluation of TCH correction training

- 1日の中で何回貼り紙（リマインダー）に気づき，そのうち何回TCH是正を行ったか？
- その時にしっかり脱力ができたか？
  全身の脱力ができたか？
- 是正訓練を行う時にわからないことがないか？
- 訓練ができない環境・条件がないか？
- こちらの指導法を確実に実践しているか？
  貼り紙の枚数は？
  貼っている場所は？
  貼り紙が景色になっていないか？
- 是正訓練を行ってみて何か変化があったか？
  以前のように全身が緊張しているようなことがなくなり，力が抜けている．
  歯を接触させていると逆に疲れる．
  口元の力が抜けた感じがする．

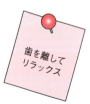

- How many times did you notice the stickers (reminders) in a day?
  How many times did you correct TCH?
- Could you take relaxation actions to loosen up the whole body?
- Do you have any questions about the practice of correction training?
- Are there any environmental factors/conditions that hinder training?
- Are given instructions exactly followed?
  How many are stickers used?
  Where are the stickers posted?
  Have the stickers assimilated into surrounding things?
- Any following changes as results of correction training?
  The whole body is loosened.
  Teeth contact now requires effort.
  Tension around the mouth seems to have disappeared.

Fig. 6-9　TCH是正訓練の評価時にチェックするポイント
Fig. 6-9　Checkpoints for evaluation of TCH correction training

- 貼り紙は同じ色で10枚以上貼る．

- 貼ったら貼り紙のことは忘れ，覚えておこうとしない．

- TCHの話をすると，一生懸命歯を離そうとする患者が多い．
  意識して歯を離すことをしてはいけない．

- 無理に歯を離そうとすると，普段使わない筋肉を使い，痛みが出やすくなる．

- 歯を離すために唇や頬粘膜をはさんだり，ガムを介在させたりする患者もいる．
  この行動自体も筋肉の疲労につながる．

- 時間が経過すると，貼り紙は景色になり，気づく効果がなくなってしまう．貼る場所を変える，色を変えるなど工夫が必要．

Fig.6-10 TCH是正訓練指導時の注意点

通常はここまでに短くとも2〜3カ月を要する．

2) TCH是正の評価法

　TCH是正訓練の評価は，2週間に一度くらいのペースが適切と思われる．これは来院間隔があくことで患者のモチベーションが下がることを防ぎ，正しい是正法を行っているかをチェックする目的もある．

　評価時には，**Fig.6-9**に示す項目をチェックして記録する．さらに，5章で紹介したLCTA（Lips Closed Teeth Apart；歯列離開）テストとLCTC（Lips Closed Teeth Contact；歯列接触）テストを用いて，是正ができているか判定する（**Fig.6-8**）．今までTCHのあった人では，口唇の閉鎖と歯の接触を同時に指示しても違和感を感じなかったのが，TCHの是正がうまくいくと，口唇閉鎖と歯の接触を同時にさせた時に違和感を感じるようになる．こうなれば，TCHから離脱できていると考えられる．

3) TCHの是正がうまくいかない時の注意点

　習慣逆転法を用いたTCH是正訓練を行っても，なかにはTCHが是正できない患者もいる．そのような患者は，こちらの指示どおりのことをせずに自己流にアレンジしている場合が多い．家族から非難されて貼り紙ができない，職場で貼り紙をするのが恥ずかしい等を訴える患者もいる．

　リハビリトレーニングと同様，こちらの指導どおりに訓練をしているか，患者にしっかり確認する必要がある（**Fig.6-10**）．2週間ごとの是正評価の際に必ず確認をして，患者が正しく訓練を継続できるよう導いていただきたい．

- Ten and more stickers of same color should be posted.
- After posting, forget about reminders, do not try to remember.
- Patients who were informed of TCH try to keep their teeth apart intently. Conscious efforts to set them apart should be avoided.
- If the patient try to keep teeth apart consciously, he/she uses muscles that are not usually used, which tends to cause pain.
- Some patients impose lips, buccal mucosa and chewing gum between upper and lower teeth to keep them apart. This also leads to muscle fatigue.
- As time passes, reminders assimilate into surrounding things. Spots to be posted and color of reminders should be changed.

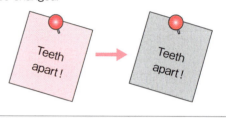

Fig. 6-10 Important points in TCH correction training

4. Evaluation of TCH correction

1) Effect of TCH correction training

TCH correction training form a conditioned reflex by which relaxation is introduced spontaneously at sight of the reminder. Furthermore, patients become aware of mild fatigue with their teeth in contact (**Fig. 6-8**). Then, the duration of time from contacting teeth to awareness of fatigue gradually decreases, and finally teeth contact evokes relaxation actions immediately. This can be regarded as correction of TCH and typically takes at least 2-3 months.

2) Evaluation of TCH correction

The effect of training should be evaluated just about once every two weeks. To evaluate TCH correction, check the items shown in **Fig. 6-9** and record them. In addition, LCTA and LCTC tests introduced in Chapter 5 are also applied to evaluate TCH correction (**Fig. 6-8**).

3) Failure reasons

Patients who do not respond to TCH correction training often make alterations to the proper instructions in their own way. Lack of cooperation with family, embarrassment in workplaces, etc. are reasons that patients point out.

Same as rehabilitation training, patients' compliance with given instructions should be verified (**Fig. 6-10**).

References

1) レイモンド・G・ミルテンバーガー著, 園山繁樹ほか訳. 行動変容法入門. 二瓶社, 2006 ; 367-378.
2) 渡邊友希, 片岡竜太, 阿部有吾ほか. 患者教育と簡易スプリントが顎関節症患者における日中クレンチングの意識化に及ぼす効果. 日顎誌. 2010 ; **22**(2) : 102-107.

Chapter 7

Patient guidance at the end of TMD treatment and management of recurrence

治療終了時の患者指導と再発時の対応

木野孔司 *Koji Kino*

治療終了とする判断基準
Criteria for terminating TMD treatment

1) 病因治療・病態治療による改善の判断

　顎関節症患者の多くは，6章で紹介したTCH是正訓練により2～3カ月でTCHを是正できる．TCHが長年あり，慢性化していた症例でも，是正までに半年も要する例は稀である．TCH是正訓練が短期間で成功する理由は，TCHという新たに獲得した癖に対し，本来なら誰もが備えている「歯が触ると離す」という反射機構を再獲得させることによる．TCHから離脱したか否かは，5章と6章で説明したLCTA（Lips Closed Teeth Apart；歯列離開）テストとLCTC（Lips Closed Teeth Contact；歯列接触）テストを行うことで判定できる（**Fig.7-1**）．

病因治療（TCH是正訓練）終了の判断基準
criteria for termination of TCH correction

- 口唇閉鎖＋歯列離開（LCTA）
  → 違和感なし
- 口唇閉鎖＋歯列接触（LCTC）
  → 違和感あり

- LCTA test→comfortable
- LCTC test→uncomfortable

LCTA　　LCTC

病態治療（リハビリトレーニング）終了の判断基準
criteria for termination of rehabilitation training

- 圧痛や疲労感の消失
- 患者自身の手指による強制開口
  → 咬筋・側頭筋・顎関節に伸展痛が出ない

- disappearance of tenderness and fatigue
- forced opening by patient's own fingers
  → no pain in masticatory muscles and TMJs

Fig.7-1 治療終了の判断基準
Fig.7-1 Criteria for terminating TMD treatment

それに対して病態そのものの改善，特に開口時痛の消失は，病悩期間が長いほど時間がかかる．それは，病悩期間が長くなるほど病態化した組織量が多く，病態組織が健全組織に回復する，あるいは入れ替わるための期間が長くなるからではないかと推測される．このように，TCHが是正できても，開口時痛は残ることが多い．そこで，開口時痛や咀嚼時痛等の機能時痛が完全に消失した時点で病態治療（リハビリトレーニング）終了とする．おおかたの症例では，機能時痛が消えた段階で，圧痛や筋の重圧感や疲労感も消えているはずである．

したがって治療終了の判定においては，まず圧痛や疲労感の消失を確認し，その後に筋や関節の伸展痛の有無を確認する．具体的には，患者に両手の指を使って強制的に開口させ，この強制伸展動作で咬筋や側頭筋および顎関節に痛みが出なくなったことを確認する（**Fig. 7-1**）．痛みが完全に消えているなら，病態組織は消失し，健全な状態に回復したと判断してよい．本来，健全な顎関節や咀嚼筋を有している者は，自身の手指で強制開口しても痛みが出ることはない．このように，顎関節症の病態の有無に関しても，TCHと同様に患者自身で確認が可能である．

2) クリックは残っていてもよい

顎関節症の特異的な症状であり，患者がしばしば気にするクリックに関しては，木野メソッドで消失させることはできず，残ることが多い．関節円板が転位してから2週間も経過すると，外科療法を選択しないかぎり元の位置に整位させることはできないからである．現時点では，確実にクリックを消失させるには関節円板切除手術が必要だが，世界的にそこまでの治療は行うべきでないとされている．したがって，最終的にクリックが残ったとしても，治療終了の判断を下してよい．

ただし，患者の不安感を払拭するための丁寧な説明は必要である．具体的には，クリックが残っていても新たな問題に発展する可能性は低いこと，TCHがコントロールされていれば関節円板と下顎頭との摩擦が小さい状態で維持され，音が小さくなる可能性があることなどである．また，多くの人はクリックがあっても気づいていない，あるいは気にしていないという情報を伝えることも，患者の不安を和らげるだろう．

1. Criteria for terminating TMD treatment

1) Assessment of improvement acquired by TCH correction and rehabilitation training

TCH correction can be assessed by LCTA and LCTC test. Meanwhile, forced mouth opening by both hands can be utilized to check for pathologic conditions including pain (**Fig. 7-1**). When absence of pain is confirmed by these methods, rehabilitation training terminates.

2) Click sound is not necessary to eliminate

Kino method is not supposed to resolve click sound. Articular discectomy is required to eliminate click sound without fail, which is globally regarded as an excessive treatment.

Termination of treatment is judged on the basis of controlled TCH and remission of symptoms. However, to relieve patients of their anxiety, careful explanation should be provided that remaining click sound has low potential to evoke other problems and controlled TCH might gradually reduce the noise.

2 再発防止のため患者に伝えておくべきこと
Essential information for patients to prevent recurrence

　顎関節症はたとえ治癒したとしても再発しないという保証はない．TCHが再度定着する，あるいは外傷を契機として再発する場合もありうる．
　そこで治療終了時に，再発に備えたチェック方法を患者に伝え，自身でコントロールが行えるように指導する．

1) TCH是正のための貼り紙
　それまでTCH是正訓練のために家中に貼っておいた貼り紙は剥がしてよいが，離れた場所に3枚程度は残しておく．その貼り紙は，あらためて見た時に歯が接触していないことを確認するためのものである．

2) LCTA・LCTCテスト
　6章で説明したように，TCHのある患者は口唇を閉鎖して歯列を離開させる(LCTA)と違和感を覚え，口唇を閉鎖して歯列を接触させる(LCTC)と違和感が消える．TCHが是正されると，逆にLCTCで違和感を覚え，LCTAで違和感が消えるようになるはずである．したがって，1)の貼り紙チェックで歯列接触に気づいた時には，LCTAとLCTCテストを実施してTCHが再定着しているか否かを確認するように話しておく．これによって，患者自身でTCHをチェックできる．

3) TCHコントロールの重要性
　TCHコントロールの重要性を，治療終了時にあらためて患者に話しておくことが必要である．TCHは顎関節症のみならず，歯科疾患の多くに悪影響を与えうるからである．歯周病に関して言えば，TCHがあると絶えず歯を揺らすことになり徐々に歯槽骨の破壊が進行する．また知覚過敏や歯根破折が起こりやすい，補綴装置やインプラント等の脱落を早める等の危険性がある．さらに，TCHに起因する側頭筋や側頸部筋の緊張から頭痛を強めたり，首・肩こりを増悪させる可能性もある．そのような問題の発生を防止し，健康長寿を獲得するためにもTCHコントロールを日常生活の中に取り入れるように促すべきである．

4) リハビリトレーニング
　病態の再発に関しても，時には患者自身でチェックをしてもらう．TCHが是正されていても，外傷や精神的な緊張から顎関節や咀嚼筋に症状が出現する場合がある．急性期は開口が制限され，機能時痛が強まるので再発に気づくが，精神的な緊張により咀嚼筋の緊張が持続すると，意識できない状態で徐々に開口制限が強まるといった形で再発する場合もある．
　咀嚼筋の疲労感や重圧感といったシグナルに気づいたなら，自身の手指で強制開口してみるとよい．再発している場合は，隠れていた痛みがはっきりと出現するはずである．機能時痛に気づいたら，早めにリハビリトレーニングを開始して，顎関節や咀嚼筋の自己管理を行う．

2. Essential information for patients to prevent recurrence

Relapse of TMD is not rare. However, self-care mentioned below is helpful for each patient to prevent it.

1) Leave TCH stickers posted

A patient should leave some three stickers posted in different places to perceive the teeth apart occasionally.

2) LCTA and LCTC test

When a sticker informs the patient of teeth contact, carry out LCTA and LCTC test to check out relapsed TCH by her/himself.

3) Importance of TCH control

TCH has a negative impact not only on TMD but also other dental problems including progression of periodontal disease, root fracture, hypersensitivity, detachment of fillings and prostheses, destruction of implant, etc. It is necessary to encourage the patient to control TCH in daily life.

4) Rehabilitation training

TMD recurrence can be confirmed by assisted mouth opening with both hands to check for pain. In case pain is perceived, early restart of rehabilitation training can help TMD to be self-managed.

3 補綴治療・インプラント治療・矯正歯科治療等の開始時期
Timing for initiation of prosthodontics, implant therapy and orthodontics

1) 咬合再建治療を安全に開始するために

現在，日本顎関節学会では顎関節症の初期治療に咬合調整を行うべきではないとするガイドラインを出しており[1]，世界的にも咬合改変治療は実施すべきでないとする勧告が出されている[2]．そのような背景もあり，多くの症例はスプリント治療のみで咬合調整を受けていないことから，TCHが抜け痛みも消失すると，咬合機能は回復する．

しかし，慢性に経過した症例のなかには，すでに他院で咬合調整や咬合改変治療が行われ，改善が得られずに来院している患者も少なくない．そのような症例であっても，咬合に全く手を触れることなく顎関節症を改善できることは，これまで説明してきたとおりである．

ただ，このような症例においては，顎関節症が治癒した後に，それまでの治療行為によって崩れた咬合の再建治療を行わねばならない．その場合，顎関節症が改善したからといって，すぐに咬合再建治療に着手するのは危険である．というのは，痛みや機能障害が消えた直後の顎筋や顎関節は脆弱であり，ほんの些細な問題で症状を再発させやすいからである．補綴治療の場合，咬合高径や咬合接触点の変化，矯正歯科治療なら動的治療の開始を契機としてTCHが再度長時間化する場合がある．是正前ほど長くなくても，筋や顎関節が脆弱な状態にあると症状の再発を招きやすい．そのため，TCHの確認は継続すべきであり，症状の再発を認めた場合は咬合の再建治療を中断して回復を待つという，治療を急がない姿勢が重要である．

また症状再発を防ぐには，顎関節症の治療が終了した状態のまま一定期間，経過を観察すべきである．明確な基準はないが，おおよそ2カ月の経過観察で問題なければ，咬合再建治療を開始しても安全だろう．その間に顎筋や顎関節の強さが増し，下顎位も安定するはずである．

Chapter 7　治療終了時の患者指導と再発時の対応

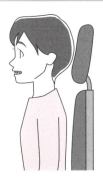

1. 治療椅子の背もたれを垂直にして，患者に姿勢を正して座ってもらう．	1. Have the patient seated in a dental chair with the backrest upright for a proper posture.
2. 視線を正面に向けたまま，細かくタッピングを行わせる．	2. Instruct the patient to perform a quick tapping while looking straight ahead.
3. 日を変えて検査しても，最初に咬合接触する部位が同じになっているなら，下顎位は安定している．	3. The same first contact point observed on a different day indicates that the stability of the mandibular position has been established.

Fig. 7-2　下顎位安定の確認
Fig. 7-2　How to assess the stability of mandibular position

2）下顎位の安定を確認する方法

　経過観察の後に下顎位が安定したことを確認する方法に触れておく（**Fig. 7-2**）．患者を治療椅子に座らせて背もたれを垂直にし，姿勢を正した起座位を指示する．その状態で視線を正面に向けたまま，細かくタッピングを行わせる．下顎位が安定しているなら，歯列中のどこかの歯が，いつも最初に接触するはずである．その位置は，障害のない顎関節と顎筋によって決まる最初の咬合接触点である．これが日を変えて検査してもいつも同じ接触点となっているなら，筋の疲労や脆弱性が消え，安定した下顎位が戻ったことを示している．その下顎位に合わせて咬合再建治療を行うことで，顎関節や顎筋に負担の少ない咬合再構成が可能になる．

　このような咬合再建が必要な症例においては，これまでの咬合治療によって，咬合高径が不適切に設定されている場合も珍しくない．そのような症例であっても，TCHのコントロールができているなら，咬合高径をある程度変更することも可能である．

3. Timing for initiation of prosthodontics, implant therapy and orthodontics

1) To start occlusal reconstruction therapy safely

Although treatments to change occlusion are not recommended in this text, some patients have already undergone occlusal treatment at other clinics. Occlusal reconstruction treatment is required for these patients following the disappearance of TMD symptoms. The importance of not scrambling to address the occlusal problem cannot be overemphasized. After pain and functional disorder disappeared, it takes approximately two months for jaw muscles and TMJ to recover from their vulnerability. This period should be used for follow-up to assess occlusal stability. TCH relapses in some patients as a result of occlusal therapies. In such cases, it is necessary to interrupt treatment and wait until TCH is corrected.

2) How to check the stability of mandibular position

Have the patient seated in a dental chair with the backrest upright. Then instruct the patient to perform a quick tapping while looking straight ahead. If the mandibular position is stable, an identical tooth in the dentition is always to contact first. The same contact point observed on a different day indicates that the stability of the mandibular position has been established and occlusal treatment based on this position can be started (**Fig. 7-2**).

4 顎関節症再発時の対応
How to manage relapsed TMD

1) まずは患者に自主対応してもらう

　顎関節症が再発したとしても，木野メソッドの病因治療と病態治療はいずれも，基本的に患者自身がトレーニングで行うものである．そのため，他の歯科疾患のような診療室での対応が必須というわけではない．

　上述したように，TCHの再定着や顎関節症の再発は，患者自身で確認できる．したがって，再発時の最初の対応も患者自身で即時に行ってもらう．TCHが再定着していたなら，TCH是正訓練を再開する．強制開口で痛みが出たなら，急性期で自発痛や強い機能時痛がある間は冷湿布で痛みを和らげながら安静にし，痛みが和らいだらリハビリトレーニングを行う．1週間ほど自主対応してもらい，症状の改善が得られなければその時点で担当医に連絡するように，通院終了時に話しておくのがよいだろう．

2) 来院時の対応

　患者を来院させて診察する場合は，問診で，どのようなことがTCHの再定着を招いたのか，あるいは契機となる外傷はなかったかといった点を明らかにする．該当すると思われる問題を見出したならば，その問題に対する対処法を患者とともに考える必要がある．

　法律事務所に勤める29歳の女性の症例で説明してみよう．彼女は，終日パソコンに向かって法律関係の書類を作成していた．初診時に右側顎関節の非復位性関節円板前方転位と診断した．TCH（+）であったため，TCH是正訓練とリハビリトレーニング（関節可動化訓練）を指導した．症状が消えてからの咬合治療の必要性はないと判断し，通院2カ月で終診とした．

　その後1年ほどして痛みが再発し，自主的な対応では改善が不十分であったため再来することとなった．こういった場合に問題点を見つけるためのツールとしても，生活・行動要因調査票（付録No.3）は有用である．この患者にも調査票への回答をしてもらったところ，通院終了後半年ほどして，職場で新人に対する指導業務が加わり，精神的にイライラする頻度が増えたこと，勤務時間終了近くになると開口障害が強まること，一方，休日は夕方になっても症状が悪化しないことが明らかになった．

　この患者の顎関節症再発のストーリーは，次のように考えられた（**Fig.7-3**）．担当業務の増加に伴い，パソコン作業を短時間で終える必要があって作業を急ぐようになり，加えて新人の教育が思うように進まない焦燥感から，TCHの再定着を招いたと思われる．これが今回の再発の最大原因と思われる理由は，勤務のない休日には症状が悪化していないことである．基本的にはTCHはコントロールされているが，ストレスが強まると歯列が接触する時間が増加していたと考えられた．

　こういった問題点が明らかになったことから，患者自身が勤務先の上司と相談し，新人教育業務を他の同僚に代わってもらった．それによってTCHが再度コントロールされ，リハビリトレーニングをすることなく開口時痛は消失した．この例にみられるように，TCHの再定着はちょっとしたことが契機となって起こりうることを銘記すべきであろう．

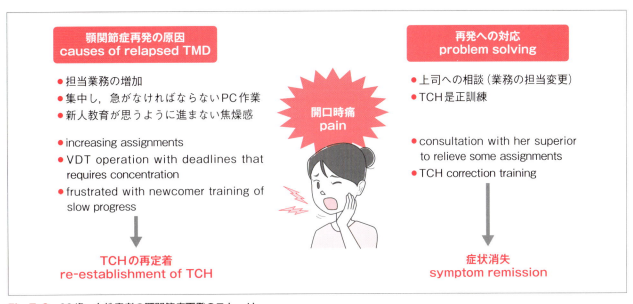

Fig. 7-3　29歳，女性患者の顎関節症再発のストーリー
Fig. 7-3　TMD recurrence story of 29-year-old woman

4. How to manage relapsed TMD

1) Self-care by patients

Patients are able to assess recurrence of TCH and TMD without consulting dentists. As soon as patients perceived the recurrence, immediate management, i.e. TCH correction training and rehabilitation training should be taken by themselves. If symptomatic improvement is not achieved in one week, consultation with a dentist is recommended. Patients should have been informed about this coping process at the end of the previous treatment.

2) Management by dentists

It is imperative to clarify the causes of relapsed TCH including traumatic factors. A questionnaire shown in Appendix No. 3 is helpful to identify contributing factors in daily life.

In a case of 29-year-old woman working at a law firm, the questionnaire revealed the increase in her assignments both in quality and quantity, frustration with unfamiliar work (training for newcomers), and symptoms worsened as working hours drew to an end. On her days off, worsening of symptoms were not perceived. As this relapsed TCH was assumed to be due to the stress of her daily work, she asked her superior to have a colleague who took over newcomer training. TCH was controlled again so that the pain disappeared without rehabilitation training (**Fig. 7-3**).

References

1) 一般社団法人日本顎関節学会初期治療ガイドライン作成委員会編．顎関節症患者のための初期治療診療ガイドライン3　顎関節症患者に対して咬合調整は有効か一般歯科医師編．一般社団法人日本顎関節学会，2012.
2) American Academy of Dental Research. AADR TMD Policy Statement Revision Approved by AADR Council 3/3/2010.

Chapter 8 木野メソッドによる治療例

Cases treated with Kino method

木野孔司 *Koji Kino*

Case 1 左咀嚼筋痛障害

Left myalgia of the masticatory muscle

患　者：43歳，女性．総合商社の経理事務職

主　訴：痛みで食事がしづらい．

初　診：2015年4月

既往歴・家族歴：特記事項なし．

現病歴：半年前，食事の時に口を開けにくいことに気づいたが放置していた．その症状は数日で消えたが，1カ月ほど前から同じ症状が再発．徐々に開口困難の頻度が増し，開口時痛にも気づくようになった．決算期を過ぎ，仕事の繁忙期が終わったので受診した．

診　察

　診療室入室時に異常を思わせる動作はなく，表情も穏やかであり，受け答えにも不安感等の精神的緊張を思わせるところはなかった．

- 頭頸部診察：左側頭筋および咬筋に圧痛と開口時痛を認めた（**Fig. 8-1**）が，顎関節を含めて他部位に異常所見（腫脹，熱感，自発痛，圧痛，機能時痛，顎関節雑音，顎運動異常）はみられなかった．
- 開口量：切歯間距離30 mmで側頭筋と咬筋に開口時痛が発現．最大開口量は33 mmで左下顎頭の前方滑走が若干制限されていた（**Fig. 8-2**）．
- 口腔内診察：咬合状態に大きな異常はみられず，アングル分類I級．舌縁および頬粘膜に歯牙圧痕を，また口蓋隆起および下顎隆起を認めた．
- TCH判定：（＋）
- パノラマX線検査：下顎頭ならびに顎骨，歯槽骨に異常はなく，28本の歯にも軽度の歯周病以外の異常は認めなかった．

診　断：左咀嚼筋痛障害．医歯大式病型分類：左側M

治療法選択のための病歴評価：受診の半年前に昇進して業務内容が変わり，仕事の量も増えたことがTCHの長時間化につながったと考えられる．その結果，筋緊張の持続から筋痛が発現したが，業務に慣れるに従いTCHが短くなり症状の軽減を得ていた．しかし，決算期を控え事務作業量が増加したことで再度TCHが長時間化し，ついに開口障害と開口時痛の増悪を招いたものと思われる．受診時の4月には若干症状が軽減していたことも，TCHが短

Chapter 8 　木野メソッドによる治療例

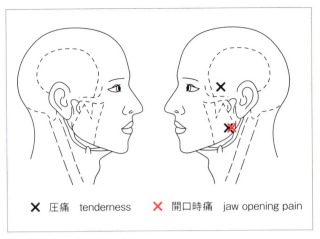

Fig. 8-1 　痛みの種類と部位
Fig. 8-1 　Types and sights of pain

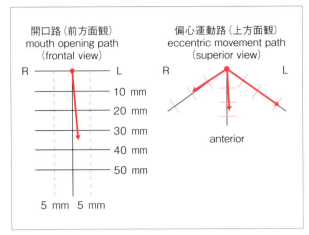

Fig. 8-2 　切歯点(下顎中切歯近心隅角部)の軌跡
Fig. 8-2 　Incisal path

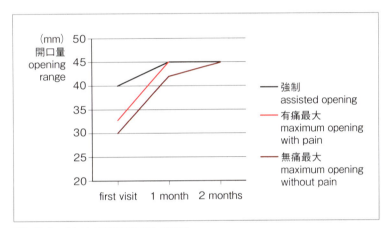

Fig. 8-3 　開口量(切歯間距離)の推移
Fig. 8-3 　Transitional change in jaw opening range (interincisal distance)

時間化していることを思わせる．

治療経過

・初診時：病態説明の後，TCH是正訓練とリハビリトレーニング(筋伸展訓練)を指導．
・1カ月後：TCHは是正されたが，開口時筋痛は若干残った．リハビリトレーニングで両手の力を強めるように指導．
・2カ月後：痛みも完全に消失し，45 mm開口が可能になったので終診とした(**Fig. 8-3**)．

考　察：多忙さがTCHを長時間化するという統計解析結果も出ており[1]，本症例は口蓋隆起等の存在から元々咬みしめ癖をもっていた可能性があり，TCHを定着させやすかったと考えられる．

Case 1. Left myalgia of the masticatory muscle (TMDU type: left M)

A 43-year-old woman visited our clinic with jaw opening pain of left temporalis and masseter in April 2015 (**Fig. 8-1**). She noticed difficulty to open her mouth in last October, but neglected the symptom. It disappeared after a few days but the same symptom recurred in March. The opening difficulty gradually progressed accompanying pain. Clinical examination showed jaw opening pains in the temporalis and masseter coinciding with the opening range of 30 mm. The maximum opening was limited to 33 mm (**Fig. 8-2**). The result of TCH assessment was positive. She was diagnosed with left myalgia of the masticatory muscle (TMDU type: left M).

At the first visit, explanation of pathological condition was provided, followed by instructions of TCH correction training and rehabilitation training. After one month, TCH disappeared but slight pain of muscles persisted. She was requested to exert greater force of both hands during the training. After two months, the pain completely disappeared and mouth opening of 45 mm was obtained which concluded her treatment (**Fig. 8-3**).

右顎関節円板障害（非復位性関節円板前方転位）・右咀嚼筋痛障害

Right TMJ disc derangement (anterior disc displacement without reduction), right myalgia of the masticatory muscle

患　者：23歳，男性．民間地質研究所の研究職
主　訴：あくびがつらい．
初　診：2015年6月
既往歴・家族歴：特記事項なし．
現病歴：19歳頃，大学受験の勉強中に右側顎関節でクリック音が始まった．しばしば開口障害と開口時痛が出現していたが，大学に入った頃には痛みが消えクリック音だけになっていた．2カ月前に就職し，その後の新人研修中に開口障害が再発し，以後クリックが出ることなく開口障害が続いている．咀嚼時痛のため流動食にしており，不安になって受診した．

診　察
診療室入室時に異常を思わせる動作はないが，不安感を表わす緊張した表情をしていた．
・頭頸部診察：右咬筋，右下顎頭から下顎枝中部にかけて圧痛を認めた（**Fig. 8-4**）．右下顎頭の前方滑走はなく，蝶番運動のみに限定されており，クリック音は確認できなかった．他の疾患を疑わせる所見はなかった．
・開口量：切歯間距離24 mmで右咬筋と下顎頭に開口時痛が発現．最大開口量は27 mmに制限されていた（**Fig. 8-5**）．
・口腔内診察：咬合状態に大きな異常はみられず，アングル分類Ⅱ級．下顎右側智歯が半埋伏状態だが，炎症を思わせる歯肉圧痛はなかった．舌縁および頬粘膜に歯牙圧痕を認めたが，他に異常所見はみられなかった．
・TCH判定：（＋）
・パノラマX線検査：下顎頭ならびに顎骨，歯槽骨に異常はなく，下顎右側半埋伏智歯周

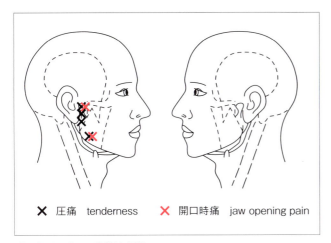

Fig. 8-4 痛みの種類と部位
Fig. 8-4 Types and sights of pain

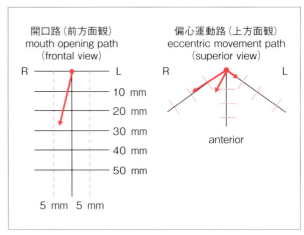

Fig. 8-5 切歯点（下顎中切歯近心隅角部）の軌跡
Fig. 8-5 Incisal path

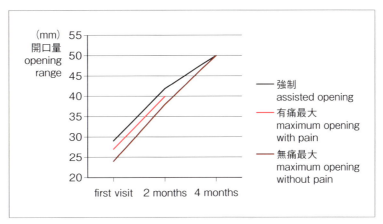

Fig. 8-6 開口量（切歯間距離）の推移
Fig. 8-6 Transitional change in jaw opening range (interincisal distance)

　　囲の異常骨所見もみられなかった．

診　断：右顎関節円板障害（非復位性関節円板前方転位），右咀嚼筋痛障害．医歯大式病型分類：右側LC，M

治療法選択のための病歴評価：19歳時の関節円板前方転位の発現は，受験勉強への不安や焦燥感からTCHが長時間化し，顎関節への負荷が増大したためと考えられる．受診の前月に受けた新人研修はかなりハードスケジュールだったとのことで，そのストレスがTCHを急速に長時間化し，TCHによる関節負荷の増大が関節円板前方転位を増悪させたと思われる．

治療経過

・初診時：病態説明の後，TCH是正訓練とリハビリトレーニング（関節可動化訓練）を指導．

・2カ月後：TCHは是正されたが，最大開口量は40 mmまでしか改善せず，開口時痛・咀嚼時痛も残る．

・4カ月後：痛みは完全に消失し，50 mm開口が可能になったので終診とした（**Fig. 8-6**）．

考　察：本症例は年齢が若いこともあって2カ月でTCHを是正できたが，関節円板を前方へ押しやる関節可動化訓練では，患者の不安感への対処，訓練法の工夫，励まし等が必要であった．それでも患者本人が積極的に訓練を続けてくれ，4カ月で終診となった．

Case 2. Right TMJ disc derangement (anterior disc displacement without reduction) (TMDU type: right LC), right myalgia of the masticatory muscle (TMDU type: right M)

23-year-old man visited our clinic complaining of difficulty in yawning in June 2015. At the age of 19, a click sound of the right TMJ appeared while studying for university entrance examinations. It was complicated by frequent opening difficulty and opening pain which disappeared after entering the university. He was employed in April 2015, and the opening difficulty relapsed during newcomer training in May. Click sound was not perceived at this time.

Tenderness was observed in the right masseter, along the right condyle and the middle of ramus (Fig. 8-4). No forward sliding of right condylar was observed. Click sound or any other findings that indicate abnormality were not detected. Jaw opening pain appeared in the right masseter and around the condyle coinciding with the opening range of 24 mm. The maximum opening was limited to 27 mm (Fig. 8-5). The result of TCH assessment was positive. He was diagnosed with right TMJ disc derangement (anterior disc displacement without reduction) (TMDU type: right LC), accompanying right myalgia of the masticatory muscle (TMDU type: right M).

At the first visit, explanation of pathological condition was provided, followed by instructions of TCH correction training and rehabilitation training. After two months, although TCH had been corrected, the maximum opening was still limited to 40 mm and opening pain and pain on mastication also remained. After four months, complete remission of pain and opening range of 50 mm were achieved, so that his treatment had come to an end (Fig. 8-6).

Case 3　かくれ顎関節症（左非復位性関節円板前方転位および両側咀嚼筋痛障害）に咬合違和感を併発

Hidden-TMD (left anterior disc displacement without reduction and bilateral myalgia of the masticatory muscle) accompanied by occlusal dysesthesia

患　者：64歳，女性．専業主婦
主　訴：どこで咬んだらいいかわからない．
初　診：2015年11月
既往歴・家族歴：特記事項なし．
現病歴：30歳頃に顎関節症（左右不明）を発症し，他院でスプリント治療を受けた．10年前には4本が抜歯となり，担当歯科医から抜歯後の補綴治療において全顎的な咬合再構成を提案され，1年ほどかけて終了した．しかしその後も咬みにくい状態は続き，何回も咬合調整を受けた．また他の歯科医院も数軒受診したが，咬めるようにならなかったため，紹介により来院した．

Chapter 8　木野メソッドによる治療例

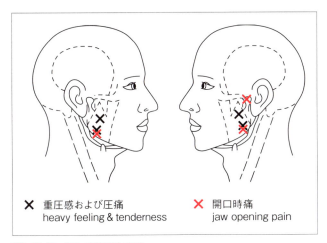

Fig. 8-7　痛みの種類と部位
Fig. 8-7　Types and sights of pain

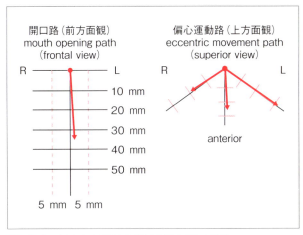

Fig. 8-8　切歯点（下顎中切歯近心隅角部）の軌跡
Fig. 8-8　Incisal path

診　察

　患者は，問診時に焦燥感をもった口調でこれまでの咬合調整の失敗を話した．性格的には神経症的傾向が強いという印象であった．

・頭頸部診察：彼女は左右咬筋に絶えず重圧感を自覚しており，触診でも圧痛を認めた（**Fig. 8-7**）．右下顎頭の前方滑走は中等度であったが，左下顎頭はごくわずかの滑走量しか認められなかった．左顎関節にはクレピタスを触知した．

・開口量：切歯間距離32 mmで左右咬筋に開口時痛が発現．最大開口量は34 mmに制限されており（**Fig. 8-8**），それ以上の開口は困難で，両手手指による強制開口で左顎関節に鈍痛が発現した（この検査によって隠れた顎関節症の存在を確認できた）．

・口腔内診察：上下顎の歯はすべてメタルセラミッククラウンで修復されており，しかも咬合調整を繰り返したため咬合面が平坦になっていた．下顎2歯，上顎2歯の欠損部は上下顎ともブリッジで補綴されていた．舌縁と頬粘膜に歯牙圧痕を認めた．

・TCH判定：（＋）

・パノラマX線検査：左下顎頭上面にわずかに骨皮質の不明確化を認めたが，変形性変化とは言えないと判断した．顎骨，歯槽骨に異常はなく，その他の異常所見もみられなかった．

診　断：かくれ顎関節症〔左顎関節円板障害（非復位性関節円板前方転位），両側咀嚼筋痛障害〕，咬合違和感（咬合感覚異常症）．医歯大式病型分類：左側LC，両側M

治療法選択のための病歴評価：30歳で発症した顎関節症が完全には治癒していなかったと考えられる．患者は，スプリント治療を受けた後，開口量が増大し痛みも軽減したので治ったと思っていたようだが，実際には開口制限や軽い痛みが残っていた．その状態で全顎的な咬合再建治療を受けたために，不安定な下顎位のまま補綴治療が行われることになり，その後も咬合調整を繰り返したことから，TCHが長時間化し咬合違和感も発症したと考えられる．

治療経過

・初診時：かくれ顎関節症と咬合違和感の病態説明の後，TCH是正訓練とリハビリトレーニング（関節可動化訓練および筋伸展訓練）を指導．

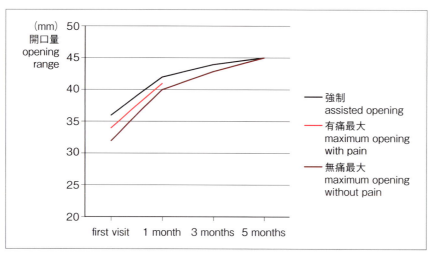

Fig. 8-9 開口量（切歯間距離）の推移
Fig. 8-9 Transitional change in jaw opening range (interincisal distance)

- 3カ月後：治療開始後，徐々に痛みが軽減し，3カ月目には44 mmの開口が可能になり，開口時痛も消失した．顎関節症は改善したがTCHはまだ残っていたため，貼り紙の交換（紙の色，形，枚数を変える）を指示した．また貼り紙に気づいた時の脱力動作を大げさに行うよう指導した．
- 5カ月後：無痛最大開口量が45 mmに達し（**Fig. 8-9**），TCHはほぼ消失したが，時折，咬み合わせを探る行動が起きることを自覚している．
- 8カ月後：咬み合わせが気にならなくなったことから，咬合違和感が消失したと判断した．下顎位も安定したので，再度の咬合再建治療を開始した．
- 10カ月後：補綴治療が終了し，定期的な経過観察に移行．

考　察：本症例のように，スプリント治療等を受けたものの，完全には治癒しないまま経過している「かくれ顎関節症」患者が多く存在している．そのような不安定な下顎位を考慮せずに補綴治療を開始することによって隠れていた顎関節症が再発する，あるいは本症例のように咬合違和感をも発症する症例は稀ではない．

本症例では，TCH是正訓練とリハビリトレーニングによって顎関節症が治癒した．その後TCHの是正に時間を要したものの，TCHが是正されるにつれて咬合違和感も消えていった．

Case 3.　Hidden-TMD〔left anterior disc displacement without reduction (TMDU type: left LC) and bilateral myalgia of the masticatory muscle (TMDU type: bilateral M)〕accompanied by occlusal dysesthesia

A 64-year-old woman was referred to our clinic complaining about instability of occlusion in November 2015. She had experienced treatment for TMD at the age of around 30. Ten years ago she had four teeth extracted. Then, the full-mouth reconstruction of occlusion was proposed by the prosthodontist. Following patient's agreement, the treatment started and took over a year until completion. However, the biting difficulty persisted and occlusal adjustments were repeated. She also visited several other dentists, but none of them could solve her problem, that she came to our clinic with a referral letter.

In the medical interview, she irritably talked about the failure of occlusal adjustments she had ever undergone. Neuroticism was pronounced in her personality. She always had heavy feeling on the left and right masseter, and tenderness was induced by palpation (**Fig. 8-7**). Her left condylar path was strictly limited. Jaw opening pain appeared on the left and right masseter coinciding with the opening range of 32 mm. The maximum opening was limited to 34 mm (**Fig. 8-8**). Dull pain appeared on the left TMJ with assited opening by her both hands, which proved the existence of hidden-TMD. In oral cavity, all teeth on the upper and lower jaws were restored with MB porcelain crowns of which occlusal surfaces were flattened by the repeated occlusal adjustments. The result of TCH assessment was positive.

She was diagnosed with hidden-TMD (left anterior disc displacement without reduction (TMDU type: left LC) and bilateral myalgia of the masticatory muscle (TMDU type: bilateral M) accompanied by occlusal dysesthesia.

Explanation of her hidden pathological conditions and occlusal dysesthesia was provided, followed by instructions of TCH correction training and rehabilitation training. After five months, her mouth opening range reached 45 mm without pain (**Fig. 8-9**). Although her TCH disappeared, she still had a light dysesthesia. After eight months, she no longer bothered about occlusal position and the mandibular position was also stabilized, that the occlusal reconstruction was resumed. After ten months, occlusal treatment finished without recurrence of dysesthesia.

Reference

1) Sato F, Kino K, Sugisaki M, et al. Teeth contacting habit as a contributing factor to chronic pain in patients with temporomandibular disorders. *J Med Dent Sci.* 2006; **53**: 103-109.

Index

あ

意識化訓練 57
医歯大式病型分類 26
痛み 10
医療面接 12
運動時痛 22

か

開口維持訓練 33
開口時痛 64
開口量 22
開閉口路 23
下顎位安定 67
顎関節円板障害 72
顎関節円板障害（Ⅲ型） 24
顎関節症 20
顎関節痛障害（Ⅱ型） 24
かくれ顎関節症 20, 74
可動域 10
ガム咀嚼訓練 33
関節可動化訓練 31
鑑別診断 20
機能時痛 64
木野メソッド 9
寄与因子 38, 52
競合反応訓練 59
強制開口量 23
頬粘膜圧痕 48
筋伸展訓練 32
筋負荷訓練 33
クリック 64
クレンチング 40
咬合違和感 74
咬合感覚異常症 75
咬合再建治療 66
咬合調整 66
行動要因 39

さ

再発防止 65
自覚症状タイプ 16
自覚症状・他覚所見乖離タイプ 17
歯科心身症 14
自主対応 68
質問票 13
習慣逆転法 10, 56
上下歯列接触癖 8, 39, 53
触診 22
自律神経失調症 14
歯列接触テスト 48
歯列離開テスト 48
心身症タイプ 18
身体化症状 17
身体疾患・精神疾患併存タイプ 17
診断基準 20
心理社会的要因 13
ストレス 14, 45
生活・行動要因調査票 68
精神医学的医療面接 12
精神科 16
精神疾患 14
精密作業 42, 45
舌圧痕 48
咀嚼筋痛障害 70, 72, 74
咀嚼筋痛障害（Ⅰ型） 24

た

多因子病因説 37
多愁訴 14
単一病因説 37
付き添い 13
積み木おろし治療法 52
積み木モデル 37
動機づけ 57

は

貼り紙 57, 65
非復位性関節円板前方転位 72, 74
病因 8
病因診断 37
病因治療 52
病態 8
病態診断 20
病態治療 30
病態分類 24
不定愁訴 14
閉眼判定法 47
変形性顎関節症（Ⅳ型） 26
偏咀嚼 42

ま

慢性疼痛 14
無痛開口量 22
問診 21

や

有痛開口量 23

ら

リハビリトレーニング 8, 10, 30, 65
リマインダー 57

欧文

LCTA 48, 65
LCTC 48, 65
MW分類 16
TCH 8, 40, 53
TCHコントロール 65
TCH是正訓練 8, 10, 40, 54
TCHの保有割合 42
Tooth Contacting Habit 8, 40, 53

TCHマネジメントとリハビリトレーニングで治す顎関節症
日本発 木野メソッドによるアプローチ　　ISBN978-4-263-44554-9

2019年 6 月25日　第1版第1刷発行

著　者　木　野　孔　司
発行者　白　石　泰　夫
発行所　医歯薬出版株式会社

〒113-8612　東京都文京区本駒込1-7-10
TEL.（03）5395-7638（編集）・7630（販売）
FAX.（03）5395-7639（編集）・7633（販売）
https://www.ishiyaku.co.jp/
郵便振替番号 00190-5-13816

乱丁，落丁の際はお取り替えいたします．　　　印刷・真興社／製本・明光社
© Ishiyaku Publishers, Inc., 2019.　Printed in Japan

本書の複製権・翻訳権・翻案権・上映権・譲渡権・貸与権・公衆送信権（送信可能化権を含む）・口述権は，医歯薬出版（株）が保有します．
本書を無断で複製する行為（コピー，スキャン，デジタルデータ化など）は，「私的使用のための複製」などの著作権法上の限られた例外を除き禁じられています．また私的使用に該当する場合であっても，請負業者等の第三者に依頼し上記の行為を行うことは違法となります．

[JCOPY]＜出版者著作権管理機構　委託出版物＞
本書をコピーやスキャン等により複製される場合は，そのつど事前に出版者著作権管理機構（電話03-5244-5088，FAX 03-5244-5089，e-mail：info@jcopy.or.jp）の許諾を得てください．

顎関節症初診時質問票

氏名 _____（　　歳）

1. 今，どのような症状でお困りですか？

   [   ]

2. いつ頃からですか？　また，始まったきっかけはありますか？

   [   ]

3. 症状はどのように変化してきましたか？

   [   ]

4. （症状に対して）今までどのような治療を受けてきましたか？

   [   ]

5. 「音」についての質問

   (1) 口を開け閉めする時に音がしますか？

   　　はい（　カクン　　パキン　　プツプツ　　ガサガサ　　ミシミシ　）　　　いいえ

   (2) 初めて音に気づいたのはいつ頃ですか？

   　　_____年　　____カ月　　____日前から　（　　　歳頃）

   (3) 音に変化はありましたか？

   　　はい　　　　いいえ

6. 「痛み」についての質問

   (1) 痛みはいつから始まりましたか？

   　　_____年　　____カ月　　____日前から　（　　　歳頃）

   (2) どのような時に痛みますか？

   　　じっとしている時　　　口を開ける時　　食事中　　強く咬みしめる時

   　　その他（　　　　　　　　　　　　　　　　　　　　　　　　　　　　　　　　）

TCHマネジメントとリハビリトレーニングで治す顎関節症　付録No.1

(3) どこに痛みを感じますか？

　　（痛い部分に○をつけてください）

　　　　　　　　　　　　　　　　　　　　　　　　　右　　　　　　　　左

(4) どのような痛みですか？

　　不快感　　にぶい痛み　　ズキズキする痛み　　鋭い痛み
　　その他（　　　　　　　　　　　　　　　　　　　　　　　　　）

7. 「あごの動き」に関する質問

(1) 口を大きく開けられますか？

　　はい　　　　いいえ

(2) 大きく開けられなくなったのはいつ頃ですか？

　　_____年　　カ月　　日前から　（　　　歳頃）

8. 「咬み合わせ」についての質問

(1) 咬み合わせについての違和感や不安定感はありますか？

　　はい　　　　いいえ

(2) 違和感や不安定感が始まったきっかけは何ですか？

　　（　　　　　　　　　　　　　　　　　　　　　　　　　　　　　　　　）

9. お体の健康についての質問

(1) 次の病気やけがをしたことがありますか？

①肩こり　②頭痛　③肝炎(A/B/C)　④関節炎　⑤関節リウマチ　⑥膠原病
⑦耳の病気　⑧副鼻腔炎　⑨顎骨炎　⑩顎骨骨折　⑪むち打ち症　⑫頭部打撲
⑬自律神経失調症　⑭更年期障害　⑮うつ病　⑯アレルギー
その他（　　　　　　　　　　　　　　　　　　　　　　　　　　　　　　）

(2) 現在，通院している病院はありますか？

　　いいえ　　　　はい（病院・診療科名　　　　　　　　　　　　　　　　）

(3) 現在，服用している薬はありますか？

　　いいえ　　　　はい（薬剤名　　　　　　　　　　　　　　　　　　　　）

Questionnaire for New TMD Patient

Name _____ Age (___ y/o)

1. What brought you here?

   [   ]

2. Since when? Do you remember any causes?

   [   ]

3. Are there any changes in the condition?

   [   ]

4. What kind of treatment have you ever received?

   [   ]

5. Questions about sound

   (1) Are you aware of any sound when you open and close your mouth?

       Yes (clicking   popping   crackling   crepitation   creaking)   No

   (2) Since when have you been aware of the sound?

       _____ yr.   mo.   d. ago (___ y/o)

   (3) Has the sound undergone any changes?

       Yes   No

6. Questions about pain

   (1) When did you start having the pain?

       _____ yr.   mo.   d. ago (___ y/o)

   (2) When does it hurt?

       at rest   opening mouth   at meal   while clenching
       others (   )

(3) Where does it hurt?
  (Circle sore places)

            R   L

(4) What kind of pain?

  uncomfortable   dull   throbbing   sharp
  others (   )

7. **Questions about jaw movement**

   (1) Can you open your mouth wide?

   Yes   No

   (2) When did your opening difficulty start?

   _____ yr.   mo.   d. ago (y/o)

8. **Questions about your bite**

   (1) Do you feel any discomfort or unsteadiness about your bite?

   Yes   No

   (2) What brought it to you?

   (   )

9. **Questions about physical health**

   (1) Have you ever had following diseases or injuries?

   ①stiff shoulder   ②headache   ③hepatitis A/B/C   ④arthritis
   ⑤rheumatoid arthritis   ⑥connective tissue disease   ⑦ear disease
   ⑧sinusitis   ⑨jaw osteitis   ⑩jaw fracture   ⑪whiplash   ⑫head injury
   ⑬autonomic ataxia   ⑭menopausal disorder   ⑮depression   ⑯allergy
   others (   )

   (2) Do you see a doctor regularly?

   No   Yes (hospital/department   )

   (3) Do you have any medicine you are currently taking?

   No   Yes (drug name   )

精神医学的面接質問票

氏名　　　　　　　　　　　（　　歳）

以下の質問について，①～④のなかから最も自分に合うものを選んで，番号に○をつけてください．

1. 今回，あなたが受診することになった症状は，どのくらいの期間続いていますか？
    ①1カ月未満　　②1～6カ月未満　　③6～12カ月未満　　④12カ月以上

2. 今回，あなたが受診することになった症状のために，これまでに何カ所の医療機関（歯科医院，他の科の医院，総合病院等）を受診しましたか？
    ①なし（今回が初めて）　　②1～2カ所　　③3～4カ所　　④5カ所以上

3. 頭痛，肩や首のこり，めまい，耳鳴，手足のしびれ，背中や腰の痛みなどの症状のために医療機関（医院や病院など）で診察や検査を受けて，「異常がない」または「治療の必要がない」と言われたことがありますか？
    ①全くない　　②ほとんどない　　③しばしばある　　④ほとんどいつもある

以下の質問は，過去1週間のあなたの状態についてお答えください．

4. 1日の起きている間，どのくらいお口のことが気になりましたか？
    ①全く気にならない　　②ほとんど気にならない　　③しばしば気になる
    ④ほとんどいつも気になる

5. 不安を感じて緊張したことはありましたか？
    ①全くない　　②ほとんどない　　③しばしばある　　④ほとんどいつもある

6. いらいらして，怒りっぽくなることはありましたか？
    ①全くない　　②ほとんどない　　③しばしばある　　④ほとんどいつもある

7. 心配事があって，よく眠れないことはありましたか？
    ①全くない　　②ほとんどない　　③しばしばある　　④ほとんどいつもある

8. ほとんど1日中，ずっと憂うつだったり，沈んだ気持ちでいましたか？
    ①全くない　　②ほとんどない　　③しばしばある　　④ほとんどいつもある

9. ほとんどのことに興味がなくなっていたり，いつもなら楽しめていたことが楽しめなくなったりしていましたか？
    ①全くない　　②ほとんどない　　③しばしばある　　④ほとんどいつもある

10. いつもストレスを感じていましたか？
    ①全くない　　②ほとんどない　　③しばしばある　　④ほとんどいつもある

市川哲雄，和気裕之ほか．日本歯科医学会誌．2006；25：63-75．をもとに作成

Psychiatric Questionnaire

Name _____ Age (____ y/o)

Answer following questions and choose from ① – ④ by circling the number that is most applicable to you.

1. How long has the condition that brought you here been going?

    ① under 1 mo.   ② 1-under 6 mos.   ③ 6-under 12 mos.   ④ 12 mos. and more

2. How many medical care providers (dental offices, medical clinics, general hospitals etc.) have you ever consulted to address the condition(s) that brought you here?

    ① none   ② 1-2   ③ 3-4   ④ over 4

3. Have you been told that "there is no abnormality" or "no need for treatment" by a medical care provider after consultation or examination of conditions such as headaches, stiff shoulder and neck, dizziness, tinnitus, numbness in a limb, upper/lower back pain?

    ① never   ② rarely   ③ frequently   ④ always

Answer following questions about your conditions in the last week.

4. How often have you concerned about your mouth in a day?

    ① never   ② rarely   ③ frequently   ④ always

5. Have you been nervous due to anxious feeling?

    ① never   ② rarely   ③ frequently   ④ always

6. Have you ever got angry easily because of being irritated?

    ① never   ② rarely   ③ frequently   ④ always

7. Have you slept poorly due to worries?

    ① never   ② rarely   ③ frequently   ④ always

8. Have you felt depressed or gloomy for most of a day?

    ① never   ② rarely   ③ frequently   ④ always

9. Have you lost interest in most things or hardly enjoyed what you used to?

    ① never   ② rarely   ③ frequently   ④ always

10. Have you felt stressed at all times?

    ① never   ② rarely   ③ frequently   ④ always

Based on Kuboki T, et al. J Prosthodont Res, 2012; 56: 71-86.

生活・行動要因調査票

氏名　　　　　　　　　（　　歳）

以下の質問に「はい」か「いいえ」でお答えください．

(A) 癖や習慣について

1. 家族から歯ぎしりを指摘されたことがありますか？　　　　はい　いいえ
2. 上下の歯を接触させ続ける癖に気づいていますか？　　　　はい　いいえ
3. ガムはよく食べますか？　　　　はい　いいえ
4. 片噛み癖はありますか？　　　　はい　いいえ
5. 爪を咬む癖はありますか？　　　　はい　いいえ
6. 鉛筆などの筆記具を咬む癖はありますか？　　　　はい　いいえ
7. 下あごを突き出す癖はありますか？　　　　はい　いいえ

(B) 日常の生活について

8. 睡眠時間は少ない（寝不足）ですか？　　　　はい　いいえ
9. 高い枕や固い枕を使っていますか？　　　　はい　いいえ
10. うつぶせ寝で読書しますか？　　　　はい　いいえ
11. うつぶせでないと眠れませんか？　　　　はい　いいえ
12. 横になり，手枕をしてテレビを見ることは多いですか？　　　　はい　いいえ
13. 頬杖をつくことは多いですか？　　　　はい　いいえ
14. 硬い食品をよく食べますか？　　　　はい　いいえ
15. 姿勢の悪さを指摘されることは多いですか？　　　　はい　いいえ
16. 長電話は多いですか？　　　　はい　いいえ

(C) 仕事や学業について

17. 仕事，勉強，家事は忙しいですか？　　　　はい　いいえ
18. 重い物を持ち上げたり，運んだりすることが多いですか？　　　　はい　いいえ
19. 細かい（精密な）作業が多いですか？　　　　はい　いいえ
20. 室内のエアコンが強すぎると感じますか？　　　　はい　いいえ
21. 会議や営業活動でストレスを感じますか？　　　　はい　いいえ
22. 人間関係に緊張を感じることは多いですか？　　　　はい　いいえ
23. 受話器をよく肩にはさんだまま話をしますか？　　　　はい　いいえ
24. パソコン作業は多いですか？　　　　はい　いいえ

Questionnaire on Living/Behavioral Factors

Name _____ Age (___ y/o)

Please answer "yes" or "no" to the following questions.

(A) Habitual/routine factors

1. Have you ever been pointed out a bruxer by your family?   Yes   No
2. Are you aware of a habit of keeping upper and lower teeth in contact?   Yes   No
3. Do you often chew gum?   Yes   No
4. Do you have a habit of chewing on one side?   Yes   No
5. Do you have a habit of biting nails?   Yes   No
6. Do you have a habit of biting a pencil?   Yes   No
7. Do you have a habit of moving the chin forward?   Yes   No

(B) Living factors

8. Are you sleep-deprived?   Yes   No
9. Do you sleep with a high/hard pillow?   Yes   No
10. Do you read while lying down on your stomach?   Yes   No
11. Are you unable to sleep unless you lie down on your stomach?   Yes   No
12. Do you often watch TV while lying on your side with your arm under your head?   Yes   No
13. Do you often rest your chin on your hand while sitting?   Yes   No
14. Do you prefer hard foods?   Yes   No
15. Are you often told that you have poor postures?   Yes   No
16. Do you often have a long phone call?   Yes   No

(C) Work/school-related factors

17. Are you busy with work, study, or housework?   Yes   No
18. Do you often lift or carry heavy things?   Yes   No
19. Do you often engage in detailed work?   Yes   No
20. Is the room you stay excessively air-conditioned?   Yes   No
21. Do you feel stressed by meetings and sale activities?   Yes   No
22. Do you often feel nervous about relationships?   Yes   No
23. Do you cradle the phone in your neck?   Yes   No
24. Does your work extremely involve in VDT operation?   Yes   No